WY 105 AST 2011

WESTERN INFIRMARY LIBRARY

GWIG6816

Successful Mentoring in Nursing

KU-508-342

Related titles

Preceptorship for Newly Registered Nurses ISBN: 978 0 85725 373 6

A practical guide supporting newly registered nurses through their preceptorship year, linked to the Department of Health Preceptorship Framework and the KSF foundation gateway.

Successful Practice Learning for Nursing Students ISBN: 978 0 85725 315 6

An essential guide for student nurses on how to prepare for, and get the most out of, practice learning experiences.

Transforming Nursing Practice series

Series editor: Dr Shirley Bach, Head of the School of Nursing and Midwifery, University of Brighton

Transforming Nursing Practice is the first series of books designed to help pre-registration nursing students meet the requirements of the NMC Standards and Essential Skills Clusters for the new degree programmes. Each book addresses a core topic, and together they cover the generic knowledge required for all fields of practice. Accessible and challenging, *Transforming Nursing Practice* helps nursing students prepare for the demands of future healthcare delivery.

A full list of titles is available on our website at www.learningmatters.co.uk/nursing

To order, contact our distributor: BEBC Distribution, Albion Close, Parkstone, Poole BH12 3LL. Telephone: 0845 230 9000; email: learningmatters@bebc.co.uk. You can also find more information on each of these titles and our other learning resources at www.learningmatters. co.uk. Many of these titles are also available in various ebook formats; please visit our website for more information.

Successful Mentoring in Nursing

Liz Aston
Paula Hallam

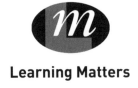

Learning Matters

First published in 2011 by Learning Matters Ltd

All rights reserved. No part of this publication may be reproduced, stored in a retrieval system, or transmitted in any form or by any means, electronic, mechanical, photocopying, recording, or otherwise, without prior permission in writing from Learning Matters.

©2011 Liz Aston and Paula Hallam

British Library Cataloguing in Publication Data
A CIP record for this book is available from the British Library
ISBN: 978 0 85725 272 2

This book is also available in the following ebook formats:

Adobe ebook: 978 0 85725 274 6
ePub ebook: 978 0 85725 273 9
Kindle: 978 0 85725 275 3

The rights of Liz Aston and Paula Hallam to be identified as the authors of this Work has been asserted by them in accordance with the Copyright, Designs and Patents Act 1988.

Cover design by Toucan Design
Project management and typesetting by 4word Ltd, Page & Print Production
Printed and bound in Great Britain by Short Run Press Ltd, Exeter, Devon

Learning Matters Ltd
20 Cathedral Yard
Exeter EX1 1HB
Tel: 01392 215560
Email: info@learningmatters.co.uk
www.learningmatters.co.uk

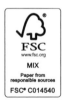

FSC
www.fsc.org
MIX
Paper from
responsible sources
FSC® C014540

Contents

About the authors

Liz Aston is Associate Professor and Lead for Practice Learning in the Division of Nursing at the University of Nottingham. Her professional interests lie in practice education and developing systems to make practice learning effective for students. In particular her focus is on the student experience, mentor support and preparation.

Paula Hallam is Lecturer and Deputy Lead for Practice Learning at the University of Nottingham. Her professional interests are focused in practice education, primarily the development and support of mentors, and clinical supervision.

Acknowledgements

The authors wish to thank Emma Celli, student nurse at the University of Nottingham, for sharing her reflections and experiences; Patricia Burr, Deputy Ward Manager, Nottingham University Hospitals Trust, and Christine Lincoln, Ward Manager at Nottingham University Hospitals Trust, for sharing some of their mentoring experiences. The authors and publishers would also like to thank Julie Teatheredge, Senior Lecturer, Anglia Ruskin University, for her helpful suggestions and comments on the manuscript during development.

The authors and publisher wish to thank the following for permission to reproduce copyright material:

Driscoll's model of reflection (Figure 2.1) taken from Driscoll, JJ (2007) Chapter 2: Supported reflective learning: the essence of clinical supervision, in Driscoll, JJ (ed.) *Practising clinical supervision: a reflective approach for healthcare professionals* (2nd edition). Edinburgh: Bailliere Tindall, Elsevier. Copyright Elsevier, reproduced by kind permission of Elsevier.

The process of evaluation (Figure 9.1) taken from Kinnell, D and Hughes, P (2010) *Mentoring Nursing and Health Care Students*, page 100, box 5.1, London: Sage. Reproduced by kind permission of Sage Publications Ltd.

Introduction

As registrants we have all benefited from mentoring as a student. If you reflect on your pre-registration programme, you will recall those registered nurses who have inspired you and developed you as an individual and as a nurse. It may be true that you have also encountered individuals whom you didn't feel were interested in you and were not always helpful. This book aims to make you the former; someone who inspires and develops expertise in others and, in doing so, it develops you as an individual and professional. Students are your colleagues of the future and you therefore have a vested interest in developing the best registrants that you can.

Being a mentor is a complex activity required of all registrants (NMC, 2008b). The role of mentor, though sometimes challenging, can be extremely rewarding. It is exciting to see students develop from novices towards qualification as new registrants, and to know that your input has helped to prepare these nurses to be effective in their role.

As stated, being a mentor is a complex activity, and this is why the NMC requires mentors to undertake a ten-day preparation programme, including maintaining a portfolio of evidence to support development as a mentor. The NMC has also recognised that a portfolio is an appropriate tool to demonstrate the achievement of the domains and outcomes required (NMC, 2008b). This book will be useful to nurses and midwives undertaking mentor preparation courses but will also be of assistance to all healthcare professionals contributing to the mentoring of nursing and midwifery students.

The book can be worked through chronologically or individual chapters can be dipped into in order to explore how to address specific issues. Activities, scenarios and case studies developed from real-life experiences encourage you to be an active student. Suggested responses are included at the end of each chapter to highlight key points and guide your development. In addition, you will be asked to reflect on your experiences or explore what is available to you locally to continue to develop your understanding and skills in relation to mentorship. Your own experiences and local systems mean that generic answers are not possible in all circumstances.

The NMC and you

All mentor preparation programmes must be a minimum of ten-days' duration, with five days' protected theoretical time, and five days' work-based learning. As a registrant you are only eligible to commence the mentoring programme on completion of one year as a registered nurse. You will be required to maintain a portfolio of learning and be successful in completing the portfolio assessment to a satisfactory standard to ensure that the designated outcomes are met.

Your development as a mentor, however, does not end on completion of the mentor preparation programme. On the contrary, this is the beginning of your mentoring journey. To preserve your status on the local mentor database the NMC requires you to maintain competence by undertaking an annual mentor update, mentoring at least two students in the previous three years, and by participating in a triennial review. The triennial review ensures that the mentor meets the NMC criteria for remaining as a mentor and that your currency, through the maintenance of a portfolio, demonstrates your continued learning and development. This action reflects the shift towards mentors taking greater responsibility for continuing professional development as a mentor.

After a period of time as a mentor you can then become a sign-off mentor for final placement students on achievement of additional criteria specified by the NMC. The sign-off mentor role applies to all students who commenced a pre-registration programme or return to practice programme from September 2007. This role carries additional responsibilities as you are required to review a student's performance over the course of their programme, taking into account all previous mentors' judgements and assimilating these into your own assessment of a student.

Moving to an all-graduate profession

Healthcare changes, and the way in which care is delivered, mean that we have to prepare practitioners who understand the need for lifelong learning, are committed to it, and have information management skills (Greenwood, 2000). In addition, teamwork is recognised as a key factor in the provision of effective, balanced care (Onyett, 1997) and there is also a need for the nurse to be an articulate advocate for the clients they are working with.

In February 2009, the Review of the Pre-registration Nursing Education Project Board approved the requirement that all nurses should be exiting education programmes as graduates by 2015 (NMC, 2009). The skills that a mentor will require for mentoring students undertaking graduate programmes will be the same, but the preparation of the graduate nurse will need to change in terms of the focus of the experience that the mentor provides for these students.

For graduate nurses to be able to function effectively as part of a team they will need to have:

- clinical and technical skills;
- research skills;
- decision-making abilities;
- ability to prioritise care needs;
- critical analysis and reflection skills;
- leadership skills.

The competencies required by the NMC will influence the mentor's focus when providing learning experiences for students. This book will help you to understand the new competencies and how to assess students against them in the relevant fields of nursing (previously called branches of nursing).

Book structure

Chapter 1 begins by providing an overview of mentoring, including the qualities that make an effective mentor. This is built upon in Chapter 2 by identifying how you can transfer skills that you already have into the mentoring situation. Chapter 3 will discuss and help you to identify how to prepare to have students, including the processes undertaken before a placement is ready to have students for the first time. It will also explore the types of support systems that can be put into place to help students to learn effectively. Students at different levels on nursing programmes will have differing learning needs and Chapter 4 will explore the level of supervision required by students at different points in the course.

Chapter 5 explores assessment in depth and looks at feedback and feed-forward to students to assist in improving their development. Not all students are the same and not all students find it easy to progress on nursing programmes. Chapter 6 will explore how to deal with challenging students. Challenging students include those who are struggling to progress in their nursing practice as well as the students who are exceptionally bright who can be quite demanding of their mentors at times. In particular, dealing with failing students can be quite stressful and part of this chapter will focus on looking after yourself as a mentor.

Chapter 7 will give some guidance as to how varying disabilities might be accommodated in practice placements. Students who have a disability cannot be discriminated against and have a right to expect that reasonable adjustments are made in the practice setting in order to fulfil the requirements of the profession and their course. However, the student still has to fulfil all professional requirements in order to register as a nurse.

For students in their final management placement, a sign-off mentor is required and Chapter 8 will explore the sign-off mentor process and the NMC requirements in depth.

The final chapter explores how to evaluate student learning in order to develop your mentoring skills further. This chapter will also explore how mentors can continue to develop their mentoring expertise in order to contribute to their continued lifelong learning.

Features

Each chapter has clear aims set out at the start, and the relevant NMC mentoring domains, and the Knowledge and Skills Framework (KSF), taken from the *Standards to Support Learning and Assessment in Practice* (NMC, 2008b), are presented at the start of each chapter so that you can clearly see which ones the chapter addresses.

Case studies, scenarios and activities are used throughout to help you to apply theory to your own mentoring experiences. You will also be asked to undertake some activities to ascertain the systems relating to mentorship that are provided locally as some systems do vary from one institution to another. Where relevant, research concept and theory summaries are also provided to help you to understand important issues.

The NMC standards refer to placements as practice learning experiences or practice learning opportunities, and the terms are used interchangeably throughout the text.

This book also contains a glossary on page 126 to assist you with unfamiliar terms. Glossary terms are in bold in the first instance that they appear.

And finally...

Enjoy your mentorship course and use this book to support the theoretical preparation and work-based learning activities that make up your mentor preparation programme.

Nursing is changing all of the time, which means that the preparation we provide for registrants in supporting their practice learning must change to meet the needs of the students. As you begin your journey to become a mentor, aim to be the best mentor that you can. Successful and effective mentoring will help to ensure that nurses in the future remain as committed to care excellence as you do.

Chapter 1
The development of mentorship

NMC mentor domains and the KSF

This chapter maps to the following NMC mentor domains from the *Standards to Support Learning and Assessment in Practice* (NMC, 2008b) and to the following NHS Knowledge and Skills Framework elements.

NMC mentor domains

6. Context of practice
Support learning within a context of practice that reflects healthcare and educational policies, managing change to ensure that particular professional needs are met within a learning environment that also supports practice development.

NHS Knowledge and Skills Framework
- Communication level 4
- Personal and people development level 4
- Health, safety and security level 3
- Service improvement level 2
- Quality level 2
- Learning and development level 3

Chapter aims

By the end of this chapter you will be able to:
- define mentorship;
- give a brief overview of the stages of mentorship;
- outline the qualities that contribute to effective mentorship;
- describe how the changing health care context impacts upon mentorship ;
- briefly outline how mentoring can be used to aid the personal and professional development of the mentor.

Introduction

There are many definitions of mentorship in nursing literature, and several different terms used to describe people who facilitate and assess student learning. This can be extremely confusing, which is why it is important for you to understand what the current expectations are of the mentoring role.

The NMC, in its *Standards to Support Learning and Assessment in Practice* (NMC, 2008b), has outlined quite clearly its view of the different stages of mentorship and what is expected from a mentor today.

You will have been mentored as a student yourself, and will probably remember really excellent mentors who have influenced the way you developed as a student and how you practise as a nurse. Unfortunately, most students have also experienced working with mentors, or other registered nurses, who have not been interested in their development. This is why it is important to explore what can enhance and detract from student learning, so that you can make sure that the environment and your approach to mentoring will facilitate and enhance student learning.

The constant change experienced by staff working in healthcare today can also be quite daunting and can impact on the learning environment. Changes to the way healthcare is delivered are likely to continue, and these changes will influence the way you are likely to be mentoring students.

Mentoring is a complex role and, like any skill, it takes practice to develop proficiency in mentoring skills. In this chapter we will focus on defining what mentorship is, exploring the key qualities that contribute to successful mentorship. In addition the chapter will address recent changes to nursing programmes and how this will affect facilitation of learning and assessment of student competency.

What is a mentor?

Since mentoring was introduced in the UK from the USA there has been a lot of debate about what a mentor actually is, or should be. The term mentor literally means a wise and trusted friend (Barlow, 1991). However, there has been a lack of agreement over what the role is, with many terms being used interchangeably to describe a mentor. These terms include supervisor, mentor, preceptor, coordinator, facilitator and assessor. Haggerty (1986) refers to this lack of agreement regarding a definition as a definition quagmire.

Activity 1.1: Critical thinking

What do you think the following terms mean?
- supervisor;
- mentor;
- preceptor;
- coordinator;
- facilitator;
- assessor.

Suggested definitions are included at the end of the chapter.

Using lots of different terms interchangeably has led to confusion over what a mentor should be. In fact, if you look at your explanation of what terms mean from Activity 1.1, there are not always clear-cut explanations that separate one activity from another. Effective mentoring will incorporate, to varying degrees, some or all of these activities at some point.

Although many practice-based professions have traditionally relied on clinical staff to support, supervise and teach students in practice settings (Andrews and Wallis, 1999), mentoring has not been seen as a priority in nursing (Miller, 2006).

The English National Board (ENB) in 1989 defined a mentor as someone selected by a student to assist, befriend, guide, advise and counsel. It also stated that the mentor would not normally be involved in formal supervision and **assessment** of the student. This definition was later revised and added to by the ENB and Department of Health (DoH and ENB, 2001) to mean someone who facilitates learning, supervises students and, in addition, also assesses students.

More recently, the Nursing and Midwifery Council (NMC) published *Standards to Support Learning and Assessment in Practice* (SLAIP) in 2006 with an amended version in 2008. These standards set out very clearly for the first time what is expected at each stage of mentoring, including the requirement that a **new registrant** must be qualified for a minimum of 12 months before commencing the mentor's course.

The NMC also defines four stages of mentoring and clearly states outcomes for mentoring that are required for each stage under specific domains. This has clarified what is expected of the mentor's role and also emphasises the professional roles of a mentor, which the next section will now examine.

Overview of mentoring

The role of a mentor has been demonstrated to be pivotal to the student's clinical learning experience (Myell et al., 2008) but mentors often feel inadequately prepared and equipped for their role (Andrews and Wallis, 1999). However, those who felt best prepared had undertaken a specific preparation course. The NMC (2008b) has provided clarity for mentor preparation programmes in terms of what must be achieved by the registrant, and what is expected of the mentor role at each stage that it has specified.

Stages of mentorship: a brief summary

Stage 1 – the new registrant role

This is the role that all registrants undertake whilst getting to grips with their roles and responsibilities as a nurse. While you are expected to facilitate students and develop others' competence, there is no role in terms of making summative assessment of a student. This role is undertaken during the first year as a new registrant.

Stage 2 – the mentor (including **sign-off mentors**)

The mentor has a specific remit to provide and facilitate learning opportunities for students and to assess the student's competence relevant to the stage of the course they are at. Mentors require a ten-day preparation programme consisting of five days' theoretical preparation and five days' **work-based learning** activities.

continued overleaf...

continued...

Mentors for first year students can be a nurse from any field of practice, or a healthcare professional who has undertaken some form of preparation, has been updated annually and is on the mentor database. Mentors for second and third year students must be a registered nurse from any field of practice (unless it is the student's management practice learning experience).

As a result of the review of pre-registration education by the NMC (2010a), there have been changes that now allow all healthcare professionals to mentor and assess students in the first year of the programme in competencies that are relevant to their own profession. This allows further expansion of inter-professional experiences for students within the type of practice learning experiences they are undertaking.

Sign-off mentors are experienced mentors who have achieved specific additional criteria that are required for a student undergoing their management practice learning opportunity in their final year. They have additional responsibilities and accountability with regard to taking into account all previous mentor's judgements using the student's Ongoing Achievement Record in order to make a final summative judgement about a student's suitability to enter the professional register. However, the NMC does not require a further period of formal training for this role but the mentor must be registered in the same field of practice (previously known as branch of nursing) that the student is aiming to register in.

Stage 3 – the practice teacher

The **practice teacher** is a registrant who has normally been a mentor and then undertaken additional preparation of 30 days' duration. Practice teacher qualifications are required for all students who are undertaking courses leading to registration as a specialist (e.g. Specialist Practitioner Qualifications).

Stage 4 – the teacher

Teachers are NMC registrants who have undertaken an NMC-approved teacher preparation programme, with responsibilities for organising and coordinating learning activities in both academic and practice environments. Teachers/lecturers are those responsible for pre-registration and/or post-registration programmes.

For all stages of mentorship there is a single framework to support learning and assessment in practice. This framework helps support how you help students to learn and how you assess students in practice.

Within this framework the domains identified by the NMC (2008b) include:

- establishing effective working relationships;
- facilitation of learning;
- assessment and accountability;
- evaluation of learning;

- creating an environment for learning;
- context of practice;
- evidence based practice;
- leadership.

Each domain has a number of outcomes that must be achieved in order to function effectively in each element. Each domain has a set of outcomes that individuals need to demonstrate they have achieved for each stage of mentoring.

Activity 1.2: Reflection

Look at each domain and begin to familiarise yourself with what is expected for the mentor role. You will find these on the NMC website (www.nmc-uk.org; search on 'Standards to support learning and assessment in practice').

There is no sample answer at the end of the chapter but this activity will be developed further in Chapter 2.

You may have felt a little overwhelmed as a prospective mentor when you looked at the domains and outcomes that the NMC requires. Many mentors feel this way at the start of their mentorship programme. The mentorship programme is designed to help you focus on these domains to identify how you can facilitate and assess learning for students. During subsequent chapters we will cover all domains and outcomes using activities to explore how the mentor can achieve and demonstrate achievement of these.

Many of the activities required from a mentor are ones which you also use within other aspects of your clinical practice. For example, consider the domain that pertains to the evaluation of learning. The NMC requires the mentor to evaluate student learning experiences and develop action plans for change in the light of the evaluation. As a registered nurse you already evaluate patient outcomes and develop action plans. In terms of mentorship you will transfer the skills you have in relation to evaluating client outcomes to a different context; that is, evaluating learning. Your transferable skills will be covered in detail in Chapter 2, but throughout this book we will show you how you can transfer the skills you have already acquired into the mentorship process. Using transferable skills to help you to develop as a mentor helps to highlight how you continue to develop the skills you have acquired and shows the importance of continuing to learn throughout your professional life.

Mentors using mentoring as a learning experience

The NMC supports and advocates lifelong learning for all nurses. The NMC requires that all nurse preparation programmes equip students with lifelong learning skills, acknowledging that *the rapidly changing nature of healthcare reflects a need for career-wide continuing professional development and the capacity not only to adapt to change but to identify the need for change and to initiate change* (NMC, 2004a, page 14). As registered nurses we are required continuously to develop our professional skills and knowledge (NMC, 2008b); providing evidence of continuous professional development (CPD) is mandatory for renewal of registration. Mentoring is one aspect of lifelong learning. The NMC developmental framework for mentorship was designed to enable practitioners to enter or exit the framework at any stage. The framework can also be used to facilitate your personal and professional development as a mentor.

Before you enter the framework as a registrant, your mentoring journey has already begun. As a pre-registration student you will have been exposed to the qualities and skills of your allocated mentors. More critically, via evaluation processes, you will have considered which mentors you found most helpful, and why. This is a lifelong process of journeying from student nurse, to stage 1 registrant, to mentor and sign-off mentor, and parallels Benner's concept of 'novice to expert' (Benner, 1984). Benner describes how you progress from a novice nurse to becoming an expert in your field of nursing and this is the same in relation to mentoring. You start out with a toolkit of skills which, through use, practice and also **reflection**, help you become skilled as a mentor.

All students spend 50% of their training in practice being supervised directly or indirectly by a mentor. This provides mentors with numerous opportunities to reflect on their mentoring practice and to further develop their mentoring skills. A successful mentor learns something from every student they support. Developing your own self-awareness is an essential mentoring skill. It requires you to have the ability to reflect on your own practice. Skills of reflection are central to lifelong learning and will enable you to adapt and be responsive to the many changes that nurse education will be experiencing during this next decade. The success of new degree exit curricula relies to a great extent on the mentor's ability to maximise learning opportunities that evolve from what will be fundamental changes to the allocation of students to their practice learning areas.

What is effective mentoring?

So what is the difference between mentoring and mentoring effectively? It is in the ability to structure what the student is to achieve during a period of practice, rather than just asking the student to follow the mentor and hope that learning opportunities will present themselves that are relevant to the student's needs. Just being with a qualified nurse in a practice learning setting does not guarantee that the student will actually learn anything (Burnard, 1988) and nor will providing activities for students to aid their learning ensure that the student has actually learned anything.

Case study: Students' experiences of effective mentoring

First year student – Lizzie

I started on the ward on a Monday morning and felt awful – I hate changing placements. Walking into the ward I wondered what the staff were going to be like. They were lovely. The ward receptionist smiled and said hello straight away. I explained who I was and she said she would find out who my mentor was. Normally I like to go and introduce myself and get my off duty before I start a placement but I didn't get

continued opposite...

continued...

allocated until the last minute so I didn't get the chance.

My mentor, Helen, was great. She introduced herself and showed me round quickly but said she had got a quiz for me to do later to help me find out where things were. She asked me where I had been before and asked me to shadow her that morning as they were really busy. I was a bit worried when she said this but it was okay. She explained to me about what the patients had before we went to them and what we needed to do for them and promised to give me a complete handover later that morning. She was really nice to the patients as well. She made them all feel special and as if she had loads of time for them – it was great to watch her cope so well.

I helped as much as I could but it was only my second placement so I wasn't able to do very much.

I was really impressed that Helen remembered to give me a handover of the patients when we had a short, quiet period. She thanked me for being such a great help with the patients. She also asked me if I had any worries or specific things I needed to achieve in this placement. I told her I needed to get a couple of Essential Skills Cluster assessments done whilst I am here. I also said that I wanted to really get to grips with basic things like feeding, washing, toileting patients as well as learning all I could about respiratory patients (this is the sort of ward that it was). I told Helen I hadn't had time to do any reading up on these things as I was given my placement at short notice. She said not to worry – she had a placement book that would guide me on what to read up on and a list of medicines that were used regularly on this ward. She apologised for not having the time to go through all of this first thing. I was told to ask lots of questions and that, if I wanted to get involved in anything going off on the ward to just ask and they would try to sort it out for me.

I went home that day feeling really positive about the placement. Helen had done my off duty to shadow hers as much as possible. I think I might get to learn a lot on this placement.

Third year student – Emma

I was assigned to a critical care unit where I was allocated a main mentor and a supplementary mentor. On my very first shift I met one of my mentors, John. He was very kind and understanding, especially as I was completely overwhelmed with the environment, equipment and patient group I was dealing with. I was pretty sure I was going to end up causing some sort of harm as I felt so under-confident in my abilities.

I don't know why I felt that way; I had never had these doubts before. I had always been fairly confident as a student nurse. I believe it was because I felt 'thrown in at the deep end' with this particular placement. I had never worked on this type of ward before so I was scared of the unknown.

My mentor, John, identified quite quickly that I was starting to freak out. I didn't even want to stand near the patient in case I did anything wrong, let alone do any form of personal care with all the equipment the patient was attached to. He had a word with one of his colleagues and took me off to the staff room for a cup of tea and a chat. We discussed my concerns and he explained I could participate in as little or as much as I wanted but he would always be there to make sure I didn't do anything wrong. He made me feel completely at ease and by the end of the shift (which incidentally was particularly horrific), I felt a lot more confident.

We worked together for a few more shifts and with that I became more confident with my abilities and settled in well. Even though John challenged me I did not feel overwhelmed by this.

Activity 1.3: Reflection

Think about the experiences of the students in these case studies. What made these positive experiences for the students, and why?

Some suggestions are included at the end of the chapter.

When meeting a student for the first time it is important to establish a relationship with them. It is well documented that the nature and quality of the mentor–student relationship is fundamental to the mentoring process (Andrews and Wallis, 1999) and that the relationship will directly influence the quality of the learning experience (White et al., 1993). It is interesting to note in the two student experiences described in the Case studies that, although the students are at different stages of their educational programme, their feelings on entering a practice learning setting for the first time do not really differ.

Several authors have identified essential attributes that the mentor must demonstrate in order to be an effective mentor (Darling, 1984; Earnshaw, 1995; Rogers and Lawton, 1995). These qualities are:

- approachability;
- effective interpersonal skills;
- adopting a positive teaching role;
- paying appropriate attention to learning experiences;
- providing supervisory support;
- professional development ability.

In particular, the personal characteristics and interpersonal skills of the mentor are extremely valued by students, which is an interesting point to note. The mentor's self-awareness and awareness of how the student is responding to a particular situation is also important.

Andrews and Wallis (1999) identify that the mentor must also have knowledge and be wise in their field of practice, with Spouse (1996) adding that knowledge of the curriculum for the programme that the student is undertaking is essential.

Motivation to teach and support students is also an important factor (Davies et al., 1994). This is a particularly difficult aspect of effective mentoring, when registered nurses do not have a choice in whether to be a mentor or not. It is a requirement of the NMC that all registrants must teach, support and mentor students. It is also required within the job descriptions of new registrants.

Another way you help to create an effective mentoring relationship is to set expectations out clearly at the beginning of the practice learning opportunity. The mentor's expectations of the student need to be clear, but also the student's expectations need to be articulated to the mentor. This way, unrealistic expectations can be dealt with by both parties with a compromise that is achievable being agreed at the outset. Borges (2004) also clarifies that the mentee–mentor relationship should be goal-oriented. If goals are agreed between both parties, this will aid feedback by the mentor to the student and vice versa. In essence, the effectiveness of mentoring relies on the partnership between both parties, a good relationship and facilitation of learning.

Activity 1.4: Reflection

Think about what you have learned so far. Which qualities do you feel make an effective mentor? Make a list of these.

A sample answer can be found at the end of this chapter.

Having a mentor is crucial to practice learning (Gray and Smith, 2000) and the mentor also needs to think about what the student needs to learn. The mentor needs to consider what will be relevant for the student at specific points in the course, and provide appropriate opportunities for learning. In addition, the mentor has to assess that learning has taken place. This will involve being satisfied that the student can demonstrate, consistently, that learning has taken place and that the learning has been put into practice.

Being an effective mentor is also about recognising when a student is unable to achieve the required level of competency, and feeling able to articulate this.

Chapter 5 will focus on assessing a student's outcomes and proficiencies whilst Chapter 4 explores how you can tailor your mentoring activities to the level appropriate for students at different points in their pre-registration programme.

In addition, the changing contexts in which nursing takes place impacts upon the mentoring process: mentors need to think carefully about what the student needs to achieve as the role of a nurse evolves in response to changing healthcare systems.

The nurse of today

The NMC (2010a) has placed the emphasis in all new curricula on generic competencies, with 80% of the programme focusing on these and only 20% being field-specific. We need, therefore, to consider very carefully the context of practice for which we are preparing students. The NMC (2010a) has emphasised that experience in the community will need to be expanded. There is also a need to enhance the transferability of leadership, teamwork and decision-making skills, as well as expecting the nurse to be able to deliver nursing care and expand their scope of professional practice. This means there are changes in the expectations of what students must achieve in their pre-registration programme. What we do know is that there will be an increase in the non-registered personnel who deliver care, so the teaching and supervisory abilities of our new registrants have to be expanded because registrants of the future are more likely to be involved in educating and supervising this increased number of non-registered personnel. The nurse is also likely to be more of an assessor, planner and evaluator of care than to be involved in delivering that care.

These changes will impact considerably on the expectations that mentors will have of students and on how the mentor will decide to facilitate that student's learning.

The NMC competencies (NMC, 2010a) provide some direction for the mentor in terms of what the student is required to achieve, both for their two course **progression points** and for entry to the register.

A summary of the NMC competencies required at specific progression points

Progression point one: The focus is on the acquisition of essential care skills, safety, attitudes and values that the student demonstrates.

Progression point two: The focus is on the student needing less direct supervision in practice. The student should be demonstrating that they are knowledgeable and have the ability to start to make decisions about a client's care. They should also be starting to become involved in teaching their peers and junior colleagues.

Entry to the register: The student should be proficient in all competencies identified, demonstrating that they can operate effectively as part of the multiprofessional team. They should demonstrate that they have a repertoire of clinical and technical skills. In addition they will be able to demonstrate their critical thinking skills, ability to advocate for clients, skills with regard to prioritising care, and begin to take on a leadership role within the healthcare team relevant to their new registrant status.

Nursing students will need to be increasingly aware of the patient's journey through the healthcare system and mentors will need to facilitate students' learning about the patient's journey in order that the nurse is able to provide leadership within the healthcare team. This means that practice learning experiences will need to be structured differently so that students can maximise their learning about the patient's journey. Providing blocks of practice that reflect the patient's journey will aid the student's understanding of how nursing in different fields contributes to patient care as a whole entity.

How blocks of practice affect mentoring

In nursing, the traditional view of a clinical practice learning experience is of a student being allocated to either an in-patient setting or one within the community. Both types of practice learning experience might be in either the NHS or the independent and voluntary sector. Following the NMC's (2010a) review of pre-registration education, the recommendations are that students are provided with blocks of clinical practice that highlight for the student the sort of journey that a particular patient who has a given health problem might follow. These blocks of practice are described in a variety of ways. They may be called:

- care pathways;
- student learning pathway;
- integrated educational pathway;
- learning journey;
- patient's journey;
- hub and spoke models.

This will inevitably impact upon the way that mentoring is currently structured. Students, as part of a block of practice, will spend time with a variety of either registered nurses and/or other healthcare professionals, who provide services for a group of patients.

Activity 1.5: Reflection

Reflect on or find out about the way that a student's practice experience is structured within the university from which you have students. You may need to speak to your education representative in the practice area or refer to documentation about the nursing programme that your university provides for you.

Once you have identified your local structures, think about how mentors do, or could, get information from those other healthcare professionals that students work with that could assist you in your assessment of the student you are assessing.

A sample answer can be found at the end of this chapter. This topic will also be explored further in Chapter 4.

Students work with a variety of healthcare professionals during their practice experience and it is important that you seek out their views about the student's performance so that their contribution is taken into account when you make a final assessment.

All students are required to achieve certain competencies during their programme, in order to be able to move on from one progression point to another. The whole of the practice experience should contribute to this process of assessment, even if it is a brief insight visit. If this is to occur, it is useful to look at what learning opportunities are available within the setting and to match these learning opportunities to the required competencies. It will take time to do this, and requires you to liaise with other departments to ensure that what you develop is realistic for the student; this will help you in your assessment of a student's performance. It is also an activity that only has to be undertaken once, unless the nature of that part of the practice learning experience alters. It is time well spent because it makes everyone clear about what the student needs to achieve within that part of the experience.

It can also be reassuring for any mentor to have the views of others who have also worked with the student. This approach will help to make your assessment more objective and also can aid the student in knowing why they are spending time in different locations and what they are expected to achieve.

Chapter summary

This chapter focused on providing a very brief exploration of the development of mentorship including definitions of what being a mentor encompasses. An overview has also been provided of the responsibilities that different stages of mentorship include as required by the NMC, with brief reference to how mentoring can be used as a learning and developmental experience. This was followed by the elements of effective mentoring, with an introduction to how effective mentoring can be implemented in the changing context of nursing.

Activities: brief outline answers

Activity 1.1 (page 6)

- Supervisor: someone who gives instruction to others and is held responsible for the work and actions of others.
- Mentor: a support and encourager to people to help them manage their own learning to improve and develop themselves. In the context of nursing, this role incorporates the role of assessor as well.
- Preceptor: in the context of nursing, provides support and guidance to new registrants to enable the transition from student to an accountable practitioner.
- Coordinator: someone who ensures that activities run smoothly.
- Facilitator: someone who helps another person to identify and achieve their objectives.
- Assessor: a person who judges something.

Activity 1.3 (page 12)

You could have come up with the following reasons why these were positive experiences for the students:

- welcoming staff;
- approachable staff;
- the ability of the mentor to be aware of student responses to situations;
- structure to the practice learning experience and written guidance for the student;
- the mentor providing activities for students to engage students during busy periods;
- a good role model;
- providing positive feedback to the student regarding their help with care;
- establishing experience and expectations;
- the staff obviously welcomed students.

Activity 1.4 (page 13)

You may have included some of the following:

- a friendly, approachable person;
- a good communicator;
- someone who can establish good relations with others quickly;
- a good role model;
- someone who thinks about what the student needs to learn and is able to facilitate this;
- a supportive person;
- gives clear guidance on what is expected from the student;
- someone who is knowledgeable about nursing;
- someone who has an understanding of the student's educational programme;
- able to be objective;
- able to give constructive feedback in a positive and sensitive way.

Activity 1.5 (page 15)

You may have considered the following:

Verbal feedback: verbal feedback is useful but can be time-consuming and, in addition, you have no evidence later to verify what the healthcare professional actually said.

Student practice documentation: entries into the student's documentation could be signed by the person they have spent time with. However, this could lead to confusion if the student's practice learning experience includes spending time with several other people other than the main mentor. It could fragment the student's assessment and make it difficult for the student's lecturer to be able to verify all signatures of assessors in the practice learning documentation.

Learning statements: The student could complete a statement of learning and/or reflective account as evidence to support what they have achieved whilst working with other healthcare workers. The student could also map what they feel they have learned to their competency statements with whoever they have spent time with signing the learning statement. This evidence can then be supplied to the mentor and taken into account when the main mentor makes the final assessment of the student.

Further reading

Andrews, M and Wallis, M (1999) Mentorship in Nursing: a Literature Review. *Journal of Advanced Nursing*, 29 (1): 201–7.
This article gives a useful overview of the history of mentoring.

Myell, M, Levett-Jones, T and Lathlean, J (2008) Mentorship in Contemporary Practice: the Experiences of Nursing Students and Practice Mentors. *Journal of Clinical Nursing*, 17: 1834–42.
This research is a useful read to give some insight into the perceptions of mentoring from the student and mentor perspective. It also helps to identify what students value in a mentor.

Useful websites

www.nmc-uk.org
The NMC website contains the most recent changes to mentorship and mentorship standards and is a really useful resource to check frequently.

www.nottingham.ac.uk/practicelearning
The practice learning part of the University of Nottingham website has a mentor resource section that contains a lot of supplementary information that can assist you in developing your mentorship skills.

Chapter 2
Adopting a lifelong learning approach to mentoring

NMC mentor domains and the KSF

This chapter maps to the following NMC mentor domains from the *Standards to Support Learning and Assessment in Practice* (NMC, 2008b) and the NHS Knowledge and Skills Framework (KSF).

NMC mentor domains

1. Establishing effective working relationships
Demonstrate effective relationship building skills to support learning, as part of a wider inter-professional team, for a range of students in both theory and academic learning environments.

2. Facilitation of learning
Facilitate learning for a range of students, within a particular area of practice where appropriate, encouraging self-management of learning opportunities and providing support to maximise individual potential.

4. Evaluation of learning
Determine strategies for evaluating learning in practice and academic settings to ensure that the NMC standards of proficiency for registration or recording a qualification at a level above initial registration have been met.

5. Creating an environment for learning
Create an environment for learning, where practice is valued and developed, that provides appropriate professional and inter-professional learning opportunities and support for learning to maximise achievement of individuals.

NHS Knowledge and Skills Framework
- Communication level 4
- Personal and people development level 4
- Health, safety and security level 3
- Service improvement level 2
- Quality level 2
- Learning and development level 3

Chapter aims

By the end of this chapter you will be able to:

- explain the importance of adopting a lifelong learning approach to your mentoring role;
- identify how some of the qualities and skills you already possess as a registrant and stage-one associate mentor can be transferred effectively into your role as a stage-two mentor;
- demonstrate an understanding of how reflection can be utilised to increase your effectiveness as a mentor;
- demonstrate an understanding of the NMC requirements for maintaining your registration as a mentor on your local mentor database.

Introduction

Scenario: Is Rosie ready to mentor?

Rosie has been qualified for ten months and works in the Paediatric Unit of the local Foundation Trust Hospital. She was asked by Bill, one of the senior mentors, to be an **associate mentor***, with him as the main mentor, for one of the new students who started on the unit last week. Rosie finished her preceptorship over six months ago, but wasn't quite sure if she was ready to begin mentoring, even as an associate, but agreed anyway. Bill arranged for Rosie to sit in with him and the student for the initial preliminary interview, which Rosie found really interesting but made her feel even less confident about the mentor role because of all the different things Bill went through with the student. After the interview Rosie told Bill about this, and he suggested she spend a few minutes thinking about what skills he had used during the interview, and then consider her own skills and how she could use them with the student. This really showed Rosie how she had already acquired many of the skills needed for mentoring.*

This chapter aims to provide you with the opportunity to develop a lifelong learning approach to your role as a mentor, enabling you to respond to the ongoing and forthcoming changes in nurse training, helping to ensure you are an effective mentor, acting as a role model and able to demonstrate clinical decision-making abilities. The increasing evidence base indicates that mentors who have continued to develop will help students justify decision-making in their own practice and begin to take responsibility for their actions (NMC, 2008b, page 17).

The chapter begins with an overview of how mentoring fits into your continuing professional development framework, including activities to help you explore how the qualities and skills you already possess can be further developed and transferred into your role as a mentor. Practitioners attending mentor preparation programmes are often surprised by how the knowledge and skills they are using every day to assess, plan and deliver patient care are some of the key skills they will be using as a mentor to assess, plan and support the learning of pre-registration students.

One of the principal factors influencing meaningful learning is acknowledging what the learner already knows and to link new knowledge with prior knowledge (Ausubel cited in Curzon, 1990).

When you begin your mentorship preparation you will be bringing a wealth of useful experience into the classroom. As a registrant you have accumulated a variety of skills that you can call on to support your role as a mentor. You may have already completed a period of **preceptorship**, and produced evidence for your Knowledge and Skills Framework Portfolio (Department of Health, 2004).

Later on in the chapter there will be an opportunity to explore your skills of reflection and to consider how reflection can assist you with planning your ongoing professional development. The final section will introduce you to the NMC requirements for you and your employing organisation for the development and maintenance of your local mentor registers (NMC, 2008b).

Mentoring: A lifelong learning process

Lifelong learning is increasingly being seen as an *essential ingredient for ensuring high quality of patient care* (Gopee, 2002). Continuing professional development is also a mandatory requirement for mentors (NMC, 2008b). As you will be aware, the NMC supports and advocates lifelong learning for all nurses and midwives, requiring employers to ensure employees have *ongoing access to professional development* (NMC, 2010a) with employees providing evidence of CPD for registration renewal. A report by the Prime Minister's Commission on the Future of Nursing and Midwifery in England clearly states that *There must be greater investments in continuing professional development* as one of their 20 recommendations (Front Line Care, 2010).

The NMC framework for mentorship has been designed to facilitate personal and professional development. Principle B states that nurses and midwives who are mentoring students *must have developed their own knowledge, skills and competency beyond that of registration through CPD – either formal, or experiential – as appropriate for their role* (NMC, 2008b, page 17). Interestingly, students often believe that all practitioners are experienced mentors and that being a registered nurse automatically makes you an experienced mentor! This is an important point that needs to be clarified during the students' preparation for practice sessions to ensure that students' expectations of their mentors are realistic. The students' expectations of you need to be realistic, as do your expectations of them. Students will come across mentors who are at varying stages of their mentorship development and, as we are all aware, may have varying degrees of motivation for taking on their role as a mentor.

Ryan (2003) in her study of nurses, physiotherapists and occupational therapists found four common key motivators for becoming a lifelong learner:

- the need for professional knowledge;
- updating professional qualifications;
- professional competence;
- increasing professional status of the profession.

Basic mentor preparation starts the process of becoming a mentor, updating your professional qualifications and helping to increase the professional status of the nursing profession. You may have come across some colleagues who have been waiting to secure a place on the local mentor preparation programme for some time, whilst other colleagues are not at all interested in attending a mentor preparation programme. It is helpful to understand what motivates an individual to learn. Knapper and Copley (1985) helpfully differentiate between learning that occurs spontaneously and that which occurs deliberately. Jarvis (1983) draws a similar distinction between proactive and reactive learning. The term lifelong learning in this chapter is used as an umbrella term acknowledging that, in relation to mentorship, you will be required to attend deliberate learning opportunities (e.g. mentor preparation courses and formal updates), whilst also being encouraged to engage in spontaneous learning through reflection on your practice as a mentor.

Watson (2004, page 21), in a study exploring practitioners' reasons for attending a mentor course, identified that being a mentor was not the only motivator for those undertaking the course. This study identified that 58% of respondents stated enhanced job prospects and obtaining a higher grade as a key motivator. Mentor preparation has almost become a prerequisite qualification for the majority of nursing appointments. The evidence also suggests that not all reasons for completing the course were for self-interest; other motivators centred on what they might gain from the course: for example, skills to teach colleagues and students using a range of teaching methods, and ability to teach groups thereby helping to develop overall mentoring competence.

Case study: Helena

I have worked in the Endoscopy Unit for over 20 years, we have always had students but I have never been interested in being a mentor. I thought, well we never had mentors when I trained and we all worked out OK. I thought the universities were 'mollycoddling' the students, that they didn't need mentors, they should learn how we did, sink or swim. Then for some reason last year my manager said I needed to do the mentor preparation training which I am now in the middle of, and I have got to say my whole perspective has changed. I am learning so much about how nurse training has changed, and also about myself, I have been reading a book about reflective mentoring and I can't put it down, it makes so much sense, it's like I am looking at everything through a different set of eyes, I've even been discussing what I am learning with my husband!

Activity 2.1: Reflection

Take a moment to consider your key motivators for continuing your professional development as a mentor.

A sample answer can be found at the end of this chapter.

You may have responded to this activity by referring to your need to be an effective mentor, the best that you can be, to develop your professional competence. Were you lucky enough to have experienced an inspirational, passionate mentor in your training? How did their passion impact on your motivation?

Amongst your mentoring responsibilities is your accountability for assessing total performance and providing evidence of student achievement or lack of achievement: this is often referred to in the literature as a 'gatekeeper' role. You may feel motivated to ensure standards of patient care are developed and maintained. The title of this book is *Successful Mentoring in Nursing.* Opting to use this text suggests you are motivated towards being a 'good' mentor. Continuing your mentoring professional development will help to improve your confidence and effectiveness, enabling you to support the learning of students, to fairly and accurately assess them, and therefore helping to overcome the issue identified by Kathleen Duffy (2004) of giving a student the benefit of the doubt.

Understanding your own motivators to learn and develop as a mentor will help you to understand why some students are motivated to behave in a particular way. The presence of motivation is considered to be essential to learning by most teachers; however, occasionally you may be allocated a student who appears to have little interest in your setting: this can understandably be very de-motivating for you as a mentor. In Chapter 6 you will have the opportunity to explore a range of strategies for motivating a de-motivated student, helping you to address this issue.

Using your professional skills in the mentoring process

Acknowledging that you have already acquired a range of professional skills that are transferable into your mentoring role can itself be a motivating experience. Stage one of the NMC developmental framework reflects the requirements of *The Code: Standards of Conduct, Performance and Ethics for Nurses and Midwives* (2008a). In relation to your development as a mentor, you will have been facilitating students and others to develop their competence, transferring the skills of a staff nurse in terms of assessing, planning, implementing, evaluating and managing patient care to 'managing' the learning process for a student. Apart from students, consider what other types of learners you may have been supporting recently. Whilst Junior Medics, Health Care Assistants (HCAs) undertaking NVQ qualifications or new registrants undertaking preceptorship might come readily to mind, did you also recognise the role you play in the learning processes of your users and carers? It would be worthwhile for you to consider at what stage in your nursing career you started facilitating other people's learning.

Activity 2.2: Critical thinking and reflection

List the skills you already possess that you feel would be useful in your role as a mentor, placing an asterisk by those you are particularly good at. You might find it helpful to map your skills against the knowledge and skills framework (KSF) (see table below).

As this answer is based on your own observation, there is no sample answer for this activity.

KSF dimension	Skills/knowledge that can be transferred into mentoring

continued opposite...

continued...

Communication	For example, my ability to communicate effectively to a broad range of patients will transfer to my ability to communicate effectively with a range of students at different stages of training.
Personal and people development	
Health, safety and security	
Service improvement	
Quality	
Equality and diversity	
Health and wellbeing	
Estates and facilities	
Information and knowledge	

You may have found this activity quite illuminating, helping you to identify how you can transfer the skills you already possess into your role as a mentor.

Case study: Julie, a practitioner on the mentor preparation programme

I have been the associate mentor for a second year student undertaking her speciality placement with us. She really is a very good student, caring and compassionate, a real team player who is more advanced with her skill development than she should be for her stage of training. She is also very confident, where I as her associate mentor am not. After her final interview I suddenly thought that whilst I had felt reasonably OK about giving feedback to this student, because everything I had to say was really positive, we had managed to work the majority of the same shifts so I knew how good her practice was and she had produced lots of evidence to support her achievement for her competencies. I thought what would I do if she was still so confident but not very good, and had poor skills, and the thought just scared me. How would I tell someone who was super confident that they were not up to standard?

Activity 2.3: Critical thinking

Make a brief note of how you could use the skills you have to address the potential problem outlined in this case study, identifying which skills you are confident with and those you would like to develop further. The SWOT (strengths, weaknesses, opportunities and threats) analysis tool below might help you to be more objective when assessing your learning needs. This tool could also be useful in guiding your students to identify their learning needs.

continued overleaf...

continued...

A sample answer can be found at the end of this chapter

Strengths	Weaknesses
Opportunities	Threats

How comfortable were you in identifying your strengths? Did you find listing your weaknesses (or learning needs) easier? Effective self-evaluation is central to developing good self-awareness, a key skill for mentoring, and a skill that can be emulated by your students. From experience of preparing new mentors it would appear that, generally, nursing as a profession tends to encounter a degree of difficulty when it comes to giving ourselves positive feedback or acknowledging when we are particularly good at something. We have a tendency to focus on areas that we need to develop; things that we don't know. It is about achieving a balance, being open and receptive to constructive feedback, and giving yourself a pat on the back when you do well. Encouraging evaluation feedback from your students about your mentoring skills will be covered in Chapter 9. It is how you use this feedback to inform your development as a mentor through the process of reflection that can be very productive.

What is reflection?

You will have undoubtedly come across the term reflection on numerous occasions throughout your career in nursing. Some of you will have had very positive experiences of reflection, others less so. To help practice to manage the increasing responsibility for practice learning, and the ongoing curriculum developments, mentors need more than ever to be creative and adaptable, maximising the effectiveness of their skills. Reflecting on your own mentoring practices will enable you to adapt to the changes. You may have noticed how even the most highly experienced mentors continue to learn through reflection on each mentoring relationship.

Whilst the concept of reflection has become embedded in many other healthcare professions sometimes through the practice of clinical supervision (i.e. midwifery, psychotherapy, occupational therapy), nursing has had a more challenging experience in practising and developing our skills of reflection. Whilst there are a number of valid reasons for this, one of the main barriers would appear to be a misunderstanding of what reflection is and how useful it can be.

Activity 2.4: Reflection

Make brief notes of what you understand by the term reflection.

As the answer to this question is based on your own observations there is no sample answer at the end of the chapter.

You may have included the terms 'time to...', 'consider', 'analyse', 'think more specifically about...' in your notes. Reflection involves you thinking about and critically analysing your actions with the purpose of improving your mentoring practices.

Using reflection in your development as a mentor

Using a reflective framework provides you with a systematic process by which you can reflect on your practices as a mentor. The framework can also be used to assist your students to develop a deeper understanding of their own professional practice. Gibbs (1988) suggests that it is not sufficient simply to have an experience, as the experience may be quickly forgotten and its learning potential lost. Based predominantly on Kolb's (1984) experiential learning cycle, reflective frameworks are intended to guide you through a number of stages that enable you to clarify and analyse the aspect of practice you wish to reflect on.

There is a plethora of reflective frameworks/cycles available for mentors to use; amongst the most popular are Gibbs (1988) and Johns (2005). You may find that some of the reflective models can be quite complex in structure and not easily remembered when first developing your reflective skills. Some models often introduced during pre-registration training are more suited to academic writing and are not so easily transferred into everyday practice. You may have come across, or indeed have been, a student who was unsure what was expected when reflection is timetabled into the practice hours. Historically many students have simply used their reflection time to study. There are, however, some models which you might find quite easy to use, both for your own professional development and to develop the reflective skills of the student. Driscoll (2000) revised his 'What?' model of structured reflection to a model that has three elements with trigger questions that assist with completing the cycle (see Figure 2.1).

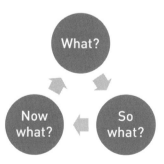

Figure 2.1: Driscoll's model of reflection (Driscoll, 2000)

Theory summary: Reflection

WHAT? Description of the experience

Trigger questions to ask yourself:
- What happened? What did you do? What did others do? What was your reaction?

SO WHAT? An analysis of the experience

Trigger questions to ask yourself: What were the implications:
- For you (personally, emotionally, professionally, developmentally)?
- For the student/HCA/colleague (personally, emotionally, professionally, developmentally)?
- For others (patients/team working/relationships, etc.)?
- Organisationally (structures and processes)?

NOW WHAT? Actions required

Trigger questions to ask yourself:
- What difference would it make if you chose to do nothing? What would you do differently if the same situation occurred again?
- What information/knowledge/skills do you need to face a similar situation again?
- What organisational/systemic changes might be needed?
- What help do you need to 'action' the results of your reflections?
- What measures could you use to consider the effectiveness of your actions?
- What is the main learning that you are taking away from reflecting on your mentoring practice?

(Adapted from Driscoll, 2007)

Activity 2.5: Reflection

Consider a fairly recent experience that involved you teaching or assessing a student, HCA, colleague, patient or relative which you felt could have gone better. Using Driscoll's trigger questions above as a guide, reflect on the experience. You might wish to use a different reflective model that you are already comfortable using.

As the answer to this question is based on your own observations there is no sample answer for this activity.

By completing this activity you will have found Driscoll's 'What? So What? Now What?' model of reflection relatively easy to apply to your past experience. Schon (1983) would refer to this practice as reflection on action, as opposed to reflection in action. Reflection on or in practice is primarily about developing your practice, increasing your effectiveness in this instance as a mentor. Helping your student to develop their own reflective skills will be explored later in Chapter 6.

As previously mentioned, reflecting on your mentoring practices will contribute towards meeting the NMC requirement for continuing professional development. The final section of this chapter will focus on how to meet the requirements for maintaining registration on your local mentor register.

Mentor registers: NMC requirements

With the publication of the NMC standard for mentorship, it is clear that the NMC is encouraging a shift of responsibility for the practice learning of pre-registration students from higher educational institutions (programme providers) to the practice learning settings themselves (practice learning providers). The implementation of 'live' mentor registers plays a significant part in this change of responsibility. It is a mandatory NMC requirement that practice learning opportunity providers are responsible for ensuring that:

- an up-to-date local register of current mentors and practice teachers is held and maintained;
- they have currency by regularly reviewing the local register and adding or removing names of nurses and midwives as necessary.

Registers for NHS practice learning opportunities are held either by the Trusts themselves or practice learning support units or equivalent. It would be useful for you to identify how and where your mentor register, sometimes also referred to as mentor database, is held and familiarise yourself with local policies for the removal and readmission of mentors to your register. Registers for the independent and voluntary sector should be developed, maintained and held by the associated higher education institution (HEI) (NMC, 2008b). HEIs must use the registers to confirm that there are sufficient mentors who meet the NMC standards to support learning and assessment in practice (NMC, 2008b), to adequately support the number and range of students they need to place. You may have experienced increasing or decreasing numbers of students in your area, but you and your colleagues are not sure how these numbers are decided. Whilst the overall numbers of student training places is decided by the Strategic Health Authority and contracted to local HEIs, the actual numbers of students allocated to practice learning areas should largely depend on the numbers of up-to-date mentors that setting has on their mentor register.

Mentor registers might also contain names of non-nurses, as one of the outcomes of the NMC Review of pre-registration training is that students undertaking the new graduate programmes from 2012 can have their generic and field competencies summatively assessed at their first progression point by a professional other than a nurse. These non-nurse professionals must meet certain criteria, which include being registered on a mentor database.

It is also a requirement that practice learning opportunity providers have in place a process for the removal and re-installation of mentors to their register. They must also ensure that programme providers have access to the register information to ensure the HEIs that the register content is accurate and up-to-date.

Admission onto a mentor register and the triennial review

Scenario: Valerie is a Community Psychiatric Nurse

Valerie works independently in the community as a Community Psychiatric Nurse and has been supervising students on and off for over ten years. Whilst she has had the occasional uninterested student overall

continued overleaf...

continued... ••

> *they have been really good and she has thoroughly enjoyed this aspect of her role. However, being out in the community makes it really difficult for Valerie to keep up-to-date with all the changes to the training of the students, and she recently read in the Standard that for her to continue having the students she needs to be on some sort of database. Valerie completed ENB 998 years ago but hasn't had a chance to attend any of the updating sessions that the university put on, so she is not really sure if she can continue to be a mentor.*

Take a few moments to consider if Valerie is eligible to continue as a mentor. Valerie's situation is a fairly common problem. Prior to September 2009 all mentors who had completed basic mentor preparation programmes like the ENB 998 were eligible to be included on the mentor databases. Different Trusts employed a variety of ways to gather this data for their databases. Therefore, Valerie's name should already be recorded on her Trust database. From September 2009 any 'new' mentor must now undertake an NMC-approved ten-day mentor preparation programme. What Valerie needs to do is to access a **mentor update** in preparation for her **triennial review** as Trusts are required to implement the triennial reviews from 2010 onwards.

For yourself as a new mentor, once you have completed an NMC-approved mentor preparation programme, you will be eligible for registration on your local mentor register. Some HEIs will automatically inform mentor register holders of those completing their mentor preparation programmes. It would be useful for you to identify your local process for registering. The details that are kept on the registers vary across organisations but generally will include names, workplace, branch, professional qualifications, dates of mentor preparation course and subsequent updates. It is an NMC requirement that all mentors on local registers have a triennial review (every three years). The review is the responsibility of your employing organisation, the majority of which are delivering the reviews as part of their current appraisal/review systems. To maintain your live status on the register you will need to demonstrate to your reviewer/appraiser that you have participated in annual updating and maintained the requirements of mentoring.

Helping you to prepare for your triennial review is covered in more depth in Chapter 9. However, you will be expected to provide evidence of having:

- mentored at least two students within the three-year period;
- participated in annual updating – this must include an opportunity to meet and explore assessment and supervision issues with other mentors;
- explored as a group activity the validity and reliability of judgements made when assessing practice in challenging circumstances;
- mapped ongoing development in your role against the current NMC mentor standards;
- been deemed to have met all requirements needed to be maintained on the local register as a mentor.

The purpose of the annual updating is to ensure that you have current knowledge of NMC-approved programmes and have an opportunity to discuss the impact of NMC or curriculum changes and any related mentoring issues. You have a responsibility to be able to demonstrate to your employer and **NMC reviewers** how you have maintained and developed your knowledge, skills and competence as a mentor. You might consider keeping evidence of your ongoing mentoring development in your CPD **portfolio**, using the eight domains for mentorship as a guide to map your learning and development. Portfolios are widely used by students to provide evidence for their mentors of how they have achieved their competencies. As a mentor you carefully consider the evidence as part of your assessment of the student's level of achievement. If you already maintain your own professional development portfolio you are halfway to understanding some of the expectations of a student's portfolio of evidence. You might also be expected to develop a portfolio as part of your mentor preparation programme.

Activity 2.6: Critical thinking

Make brief notes of what you understand a portfolio is and identify some of the different types of evidence you might include to demonstrate you are meeting the outcomes for one of the eight domains.

A sample answer can be found at the end of this chapter.

A virtual sample of a portfolio can be found at www.nottingham.ac.uk/nursing/practice/mentors.

Chapter summary

This chapter has highlighted the importance of all mentors adopting a lifelong learning approach to their development as a mentor. The activities have provided an opportunity for you to clarify the professional skills you already possess which are transferable into your role as a mentor, and identify areas for your future development. An overview of reflection has been given and a framework for practice has been suggested. The NMC requirements relating to mentor registers have been clarified with the opportunity for you to explore local register protocols.

Activities: brief outline answers

Activity 2.1 (page 21)

Your answer may include some of the following suggestions:

*   to develop your teaching and assessing skills;
*   to learn how to complete the student's documentation;
*   for the qualification;
*   part of your degree pathway;
*   to increase your confidence;
*   to learn what students can and cannot do.

Activity 2.3 (page 23)

Your answer may have included using some of the following strategies:

*   Consider why a student might present as overconfident, even though her skills are not up to standard.
*   From the beginning of the practice learning experience use your interpersonal skills to practise giving constructive feedback.

- Practise giving feedback to your colleagues.
- Give the student feedback immediately following a learning experience.
- Make sure that you give continuous feedback so the student is not surprised by what you have to say.
- If your HEI has guidance on the levels students need to achieve, you need to think about these in relation to the student and show these to the student, stating why you feel they have not achieved this level.

Activity 2.6 (page 29)

McMullan et al. (2003) suggest that a portfolio is *a collection of evidence, usually in the written form, of both the products and processes of learning. It attests to achievement and personal and professional development, by providing critical analysis on its contents.*

Your answer might include some of the following types of portfolio evidence:

- a programme of learning opportunities you have identified that are available to students during their practice learning experience with you;
- an induction/orientation pack that you have developed with colleagues;
- evidence of having attended a mentor update;
- a reflection on a particular experience you may have had with a student;
- thank-you cards or letters from a student.

Further reading

NMC (2008) *Standards to Support Learning and Assessment in Practice: NMC Standards for Mentors, Practice Teachers and Teachers,* 2nd edn. London: Nursing and Midwifery Council.
This document is essential reading for all mentors, for use as a reference for their continuing development as a mentor and in preparation for triennial reviews. The document is no longer available as a hard copy but can be downloaded from the NMC website, www.nmc-uk.org.

Quinn, F and Hughes, S (2007) *Quinn's Principles and Practice of Nurse Education,* 5th edn. London: Nelson Thornes.
This text provides mentors with clear and comprehensive guidance on many aspects of developing facilitation of learning skills.

Useful website

www.alps-cetl.ac.uk
This site has a number of useful links to resources and publications on the assessment of practice learning.

Chapter 3
Preparing for students

NMC mentor domains and the KSF

This chapter maps to the following NMC mentor domains from the *Standards to Support Learning and Assessment in Practice* (NMC, 2008b) and the NHS Knowledge and Skills Framework.

NMC mentor domains

1. Establishing effective working relationships
Demonstrate effective relationship building skills to support learning, as part of a wider inter-professional team, for a range of students in both theory and academic learning environments.

2. Facilitation of learning
Facilitate learning for a range of students, within a particular area of practice where appropriate, encouraging self-management of learning opportunities and providing support to maximise individual potential.

5. Creating an environment for learning
Create an environment for learning where practice is valued and developed that provides appropriate professional and inter-professional learning opportunities and support for learning to maximise achievement for individuals.

6. Context of practice
Support learning within a context of practice that reflects healthcare and educational policies, managing change to ensure that particular professional needs are met within a learning environment that also supports practice development.

NHS Knowledge and Skills Framework
- Communication level 4
- Personal and people development level 4
- Health, safety and security level 3
- Quality level 2
- Learning and development level 3

Chapter aims

By the end of this chapter you will be able to:

- describe the importance of the educational audit process;
- discuss the elements that contribute towards a good learning environment;
- explain what a patient pathway is;
- discuss the importance of planning the student's experience;
- explain the importance of establishing realistic expectations with students;
- discuss the importance of support systems for students and mentors.

Introduction

When preparing to have students it is important to consider the practice experience that you have to offer. Being organised in terms of the student experience makes it easier for you as mentor to facilitate the student's learning and assess their achievement of competencies. It is useful when preparing for students to involve everyone in this process; this way, you will have some consensus regarding what you need to provide for students and what you, as a team, expect from them. This also helps make it clear to the student what is expected of them and what they can realistically hope to achieve. Successful preparation for having students is measured through the process of educational audit.

The educational audit process

In managing practice-focused learning, there is a requirement that educational audit is undertaken at least once every two years (NMC, 2004a). These audits help to confirm that adequate numbers of mentors and other resources are available to support students during their practice experience. It also helps to ensure that education staff from the university and practice environment maintain effective partnerships in providing a quality learning environment for students. Systems of audit vary across the country; some universities implement an annual audit, some a bi-annual audit, and some use computerised systems which continually assess the risk in a learning environment and review this annually.

The university has the responsibility for implementing and organising education audit systems. Most universities employ a partnership approach to their audit systems, involving both lecturing staff and senior staff from practice. The audit forms part of the quality assurance procedures to ensure that students have appropriate education opportunities that will enable them to achieve the competencies required by the NMC. Without a successful educational audit, practice learning settings cannot have students allocated to them.

The preparation for an audit and the system of its implementation may vary, but the actual educational requirements will be the same, irrespective of the systems used.

These include:

- ensuring that practice learning settings provide a safe environment in which to learn;
- there are appropriate learning opportunities for students within the setting;
- there is evidence of appropriate support for students in the setting;
- students have appropriately prepared and updated mentors to provide professional support and assessment;
- care provided needs to reflect person-centred care, reflecting the rights of the clients.

Activity 3.1: Decision-making

Look at the educational audit document by your local university and find out how the university system is organised (your university education representative or your practice learning setting manager can help you in this activity).

Think about the responsibilities you have to consider when providing practice learning opportunities for pre-registration students.

A sample answer can be found at the end of this chapter.

Activity 3.2: Decision-making

Now that you have identified the key educational elements required for your educational audit, find out what is available in your area in order to fulfil audit requirements. Are there any areas of deficit or aspects that could be improved? How could you begin to address these?

There is no sample answer provided at the end of the chapter.

The key function of educational audit is to ensure that the practice learning environment is conducive to student learning and that there are enough suitably qualified mentors to facilitate and assess student learning and achievement.

Feedback from the educational audit also provides you with the opportunity to view your learning environment in a more objective manner, as the students in your setting are also given the opportunity to comment on the sort of practice experience you are providing for them. Recommendations from the audit also help you to identify what you are doing that is good and how you can improve the learning environment. Knowing which elements contribute towards establishing a good learning environment help you to measure the quality of the experience you are providing for your students.

What makes a good learning environment?

Melia (1987) described the importance of the socialisation processes of nurses, describing 'getting the work done', 'learning the rules' and 'fitting in' as key strategies used by students in order to survive in clinical practice. Feeling part of the nursing team is a key factor in students feeling that they fit in and they are then able to learn. Levett-Jones and Lathlean (2008) identify that the need to fit in and be accepted is just as pertinent today.

Research summary

'Belongingness: A prerequisite for students' clinical learning' (Levett-Jones and Lathlean, 2008)

This is a research article that describes the qualitative phase of a mixed methodology national study which explored the student experience of belongingness in clinical practice. Their definition of belongingness is the degree to which an individual student feels secure, connected and how much their values are in harmony with those of the group that they are in.

Research questions were asked of third year students which explored:
- which factors impacted on the student's experience of belongingness;
- what the consequences were of nursing students' experience of belongingness in clinical practice.

In-depth semi-structured interviews were conducted on 18 volunteers from students who had completed an on-line questionnaire. The interviews were taped and transcribed. Thematic analysis was then used to identify emerging themes from the data.

Findings

Four main themes emerged from the data. These were motivation to learn, self-directed learning, anxiety (a barrier to learning), and confidence to ask questions.

- Motivation to learn: students stated that if they felt welcome and felt as if they fitted in on a practice learning opportunity, they were much more motivated to learn, ask questions and were in a better frame of mind to learn.
- Self-directed learning: if students felt secure in the practice learning setting and accepted, they were able to make the most of their learning opportunities and felt more able to articulate their learning needs.
- Anxiety: a number of students found that if they were fearful of making mistakes or saying something foolish this impeded their learning whereas if they felt comfortable and accepted, they can relax and get on with learning.
- Confidence to ask questions: if students felt welcomed they were more able to ask questions if they felt that their questions would be answered respectfully and patiently. If students did not receive favourable responses to questions they felt it impeded the development of critical thinking skills and stopped them from testing out tentative ideas and thoughts as they didn't want to make mistakes in front of staff.

This study demonstrates the importance of the need for strategies that enhance student belongingness and social wellbeing so that the student can direct their energy and attention towards learning to care for patients. There is a need for managers and mentors in practice learning settings to examine their learning environment in order to facilitate the student experience of belongingness in order to enhance the student's development.

Levett-Jones and Lathlean's study is an important one in terms of providing an environment that is conducive to learning, but how do you know that you are creating a sense of belonging in a student? The perceptions you and your peers have about how much you set students at ease and make them feel welcome might be quite different from the students' perceptions. Mentors often do not appreciate how much in awe the students can be of them, and how they come across to students.

Activity 3.3: Reflection

Think about the four key themes that emerged from Levett-Jones and Lathlean's study. You might wish to talk to the students in your practice learning setting or observe how your colleagues deal with students allocated to them.

To what extent do you and the other staff in your area:

- welcome students to the setting;
- include the student in setting and social activities at work;
- encourage students to ask questions?

There is no sample answer provided for this activity at the end of the chapter.

Feedback from the students' practice learning experience evaluations can provide you with feedback regarding this and is developed in more detail in Chapter 9. If students describe the team as friendly, approachable and keen to teach students, this is valuable feedback in terms of how comfortable the students feel when learning in your practice learning environment. Student evaluation of practice is an important activity in evaluating the effectiveness of your learning environment, will give you feedback about how structured the learning environment is, and will give you feedback on how effectively the student has managed to access learning opportunities available in your area.

Mapping learning opportunities

One way in which you can help to provide some consistency in your approach to providing good learning opportunities for students is to identify what experiences you can provide that will enable students to achieve their competencies. Whilst aspects such as confidentiality and record-keeping may be universal to all settings that students visit, there are also quite diverse opportunities with respect to the type of nursing provided in a specific setting. Mapping learning opportunities in your setting to the NMC competencies (NMC, 2010a) that students have to achieve may sound like a lot of work but, once completed, it only needs to be amended as the care you provide to service users changes.

Activity 3.4: Decision-making

NMC domain: Nursing practice and decision-making

Competence 5: All nurses must recognise and interpret signs of normal and changing health, distress or capability and act promptly to maintain or improve the health and safety of others.

Think about the learning opportunities that are available in your setting which would enable the student to achieve and demonstrate competence in this aspect of nursing. You will need to think about what you would expect from a first, second and third year student, as you will be looking for development in the student from being directly supervised to acting fairly independently, referring to you as a mentor only to check they have chosen the correct course of action.

There is no sample answer at the end of this chapter as the experiences you offer will be individual to your area. You may wish to discuss your answer with other more experienced mentors in your area to ensure that your expectations of students are realistic.

Undertaking a mapping exercise also helps to provide some assessment reliability between mentors within your area. If mentors have a benchmark standard regarding what students need to achieve at a particular level on their course, there is more objectivity included in assessment processes and it is easier to identify whether a student is underachieving or exceeding normal expectations. This is particularly important if you are using learning pathways where several healthcare professionals might be contributing evidence to the mentor about what the student has achieved and at what level.

Learning pathways

It is really useful for the student to experience the pathway that the patient experiences during their journey through the healthcare system as advocated by the NMC (2010a). As it is not always possible for the student to follow a single patient through the whole of their healthcare journey, it is useful to think about how you can provide some insight into the patient's experience for a student. For the student to gain an overall picture in terms of the healthcare patients receive, it helps students to see how each part of the healthcare system fits together and the importance of effective communication between each party.

You need to think about structuring a learning pathway. If the student only spends a few days in different departments related to your specialty, they won't have an opportunity to develop expertise in anything. In addition, it can be rather fragmented in terms of mentoring and assessing students. You need to balance the experiences you can offer with ensuring that the student is able to develop and practise their learning in order to gain confidence and competence in delivering care. The learning pathway that you structure for a student may also be influenced by whether the student is a junior or senior student as well as by the length of the student's practice learning experience.

Sample learning pathway for a person who has respiratory disease

Student practice learning experience: ten weeks – second year student.

Weeks 1–5

In-patient experience with the primary mentor to:
- settle into the practice learning area;
- review the student's action plan and identify learning objectives for current practice learning;
- begin to assess the student's essential care skills, communication ability, confidence and ability to deliver safe and effective care and initiative in utilising learning opportunities effectively;
- give feedback on performance and identify actions to improve performance.

Week 6

May include one of the following.

1. Attached to hospital-based respiratory nurse specialist:
   - review student achievement and identify action plan;
   - attend out-patient clinic;
   - observe and participate in patient assessments;
   - observe and participate in specific interventions.
2. Attached to Community Matron for respiratory care:
   - review student achievement and identify action plan;
   - attend pulmonary rehabilitation classes for patients;
   - visit patients at home to explore their coping mechanisms in the patient's own environment and support provided in the community both prior to and following a hospital admission.
3. Attached to Practice Nurse in health centre:
   - review student achievement and identify action plan;
   - participate in respiratory consultations;
   - focus on health promotion strategies in relation to respiratory care.

Weeks 7–10

In-patient experience with the primary mentor to:
- review student achievement for whole practice learning;
- observe student performance in care delivery, noting how they incorporate their learning from other parts of the pathway into their decision-making, approach and care of patients;
- review student evidence to support practice achievement;
- make final assessments.

It is important to note that if this practice learning is immediately before a progression point the student will need four weeks with the primary mentor for progression points 1 and 2, and 12 weeks with the primary mentor before entry to the register (NMC, 2010).

A key element of a learning pathway for students is to ensure that you put mechanisms in place that will enable all staff involved in supervising the student to communicate with each other. This doesn't necessarily have to be direct verbal communication. Written statements on the student's performance and behaviour are just as useful.

When you are developing learning pathways for students it is useful to identify before allocating students to a pathway, in consultation with all relevant staff, which competencies will be focused on during specific parts of the pathway. You can then decide on how each mentor will communicate how the student has transferred skills from one area to another, and the skills the student has gained whilst in each part of the pathway. Communicating the student's achievements enables the primary mentor to incorporate the whole of the student's experience into the final assessment.

Planning for having your student

Once you have been allocated a student you need to think about the student's level on the course, as this will help to focus you on what the student needs to achieve whilst you are mentoring them. It is really important that you understand the programme the student is undertaking as this needs to guide your planning. Your mentor course will provide you with an overview of the curriculum your local university delivers, but courses change over time and you need to make the most of your education representative from the university in order to keep up-to-date with the changes that take place on their courses. You will also be guided by the competencies the students need to achieve that are set by the NMC (2010). It is also useful to consider the inter-professional learning opportunities that you may be able to offer, either through learning together with other healthcare students or by shadowing another healthcare professional (this is dealt with in more detail in Chapter 9).

The student: what you can expect from them

You can expect the student to contact the setting before they actually start the practice learning experience. This is especially useful if, as their allocated mentor, you can select a time when you are available to meet them.

Activity 3.5: Decision-making

What sort of things do you feel it would be important to cover with the student during their pre-practice learning visit?

A sample answer can be found at the end of this chapter.

It is useful to make a list of things that need to be discussed at this pre-practice learning visit so that all your staff are aware of what needs to be included. If you are not available to see your student personally you need to be aware of what has been covered by other staff members. This helps to prevent any misconceptions by the student and will help to ensure the student knows what to expect on their first day. Being prepared for what to expect can help to reduce a student's anxiety about commencing practice learning. The student orientation and learning packs are particularly important in helping to guide a student's learning, giving guidance not just for the student but for all mentors as well.

Student orientation and learning packs

Facilitation of learning includes planning relevant experiences for students, providing support and assessing clinical performance (Mallik and Aylott, 2005), with the best learning experiences being those that are planned well in advance (Papp et al., 2003). Developing a student learning pack is one way to achieve this and to help develop the student's sense of belonging to the practice learning area. Perhaps you can use the research on belongingness to guide the development of the pack.

When developing a student learning pack for your setting it is useful to decide, as a team, what you can offer students and what you expect the student to get out of the experience. Keep the pack simple: outline what all students need to learn as a minimum, and then consider some indicators for students who can and want to go beyond the minimum required at their level on the course. This guidance is particularly useful for the student as it shows what your expectations are of them. Some universities use specific 'skills escalators', which provide statements about the level of practice the student needs to achieve at specific points in the course. Do be careful of expecting too much from students as this can cause a reduction in performance by increasing anxiety and stress levels.

Case study: Third year student: Emma's experience in critical care – too high expectations

During my first shift with Sarah she asked me to go through the types of things that I had done while I was with John (my other mentor). We then looked at my action plan that I had written [sometimes called learning contracts]. She decided I was not progressing at a rate she would expect from a third year student nurse and that I should be participating more. She then set about testing me on all the equipment that the patient we were caring for on that particular day was attached to and describing the anatomy and physiological processes that were occurring. Even though I felt I was answering her questions correctly I felt that the answers were not good enough and she would continue to ask further questions until, in the end, I simply told her I didn't know. She then seemed to take great pleasure in telling me the correct answer (which didn't seem to be far from the answer I had already given). By the end of the shift, Sarah had given me homework on anatomy and physiology of the respiratory system and the ventilation package used by staff nurses on the unit. She told me to go home and revise these and that I would be tested on them the following day.

This routine continued for two more weeks. Every day my contact with patients seemed to get less and less and the time I spent in the resource room increased. I became so disheartened by the placement and I considered asking to be moved to another placement or going off sick and making the time up on another placement. Whenever I was asked questions, even if I knew the answer, I found myself saying that I didn't

continued overleaf...

continued...

> *know just so that I could avoid the constant barrage of questions. I don't know whether this infuriated her but it seemed she wasn't bothered by my development, especially as she didn't relate the work to my action plan that I had developed for this placement, which included breaking bad news to patients. I was so tired and close to tears when I tried to explain to my mentor that I wanted to concentrate on the doing of nursing and my action plan, not on becoming a fully fledged critical care nurse.*

Emma's experience demonstrates quite clearly how putting too much pressure on a student can result in poorer performance when the aim of clinical practice learning experience is to increase the student's professional competence, confidence, independence and self-directedness. It is really important to think about what you include in the student learning pack and to ensure that it is realistic and achievable for students.

Activity 3.6: Decision-making

Review the student learning pack that you have in your setting or, if you haven't already got a student learning pack, think about what you might consider useful to put into a learning pack.

Whilst reviewing or developing a student learning pack, consider the following:

- Are your expectations realistic?
- How will/do the activities assist the student's learning?
- How will/do the activities help to develop the student's professional competence?
- How does the content help the student to meet the aims of their course?

You may find it useful to talk to your practice learning education representative to check out your ideas and conclusions.

There is no sample answer at the end of the chapter.

Planning learning experiences for students can be complex when you are in a clinical environment where unplanned situations often arise (Chan, 2001). This, together with limited time within your practice learning area, means that students need to utilise their time in your setting effectively and they will need feedback on how they are progressing and what they can do to improve their performance.

Expectations of students and mentors

Key roles you will undertake as a mentor involve negotiating the student's learning, giving feedback and developing action plans/learning contracts with the student to help increase their confidence and competence. You will be expected to give the student regular informal feedback so they have an indication of how they are meeting your expectations. In addition to this, you need to provide formal feedback to the students through a preliminary, intermediate and final interview.

The preliminary interview is a chance to get to know the student and talk about their objectives during their time with you. This is a good opportunity to ensure that the student's objectives are realistic and can be met during their period of time with you.

You also need to review their Ongoing Achievement Record as there will be indicators from previous mentors on aspects that the student needs to develop. This interview should give you a good foundation to work from with the student and will provide the basis for future interviews, especially if you set a clear action plan/learning contract for the student for the first part of their practice learning experience. You must remember to record everything clearly within the student's documentation. It is so easy to forget what has been discussed and agreed. In addition, you need the written evidence on how you planned to proceed with the student as the audit trail of learning. At the preliminary interview you can outline the support systems in place within your environment to enhance the student's learning.

Support systems for students and mentors

As the mentor you are the main support person for the student, but you can also use other members of the team to help in the student's development. Other support for the student can include other registered nurses, healthcare support workers, senior students, your education representative and other healthcare professionals.

Activity 3.7: Team working

Think about how other members of the team might help to support you in developing the confidence and competence of the student. Remember to think about the support that the following people might be able to offer to your student:

- registered nurses;
- healthcare support workers;
- students;
- education representative;
- other healthcare professionals.

A sample answer can be found at the end of this chapter.

Utilising other members of the team will not only assist and support you as a mentor but will also enrich the student's learning experience through providing other role models to complement the role model you are providing to the student. Role modelling has a major influence on the observer's behaviour and students tend to take on behaviours from a number of role models to contribute to the development of the healthcare professional that they aspire to be. A student's confidence and competence tend to improve if they are supervised appropriately by a good role model (Donaldson and Carter, 2005). A key point here is that if you are using others to help to support your student, you need to be satisfied that the other staff you are using are able to function well in the support that you want them to provide and that they are aware that they need to feed back to you on how the student has performed.

The other registered nurses you use may be new registrants or mentors. If it is a new registrant, you will need to ensure that they are aware of the action plan you have developed for the student so that they can continue to work towards the same aims as yourself.

If you are enlisting the help of healthcare support workers you need to satisfy yourself that they are capable of helping the student to learn specific activities and that their own care delivery is of a safe and effective standard. You may need to prepare the support workers for this role so that they realise the importance of the role you are asking them to undertake.

Aston and Molassiotis (2003) describe the preparation that both senior and junior students undergo in order to make the most of peer support learning. Using senior students to assist junior students to develop their clinical practice benefits the senior students as much as the junior ones. It is a great motivator to learn, and helps the senior student to ensure that their own practice is of a high standard. However, if you are using senior students to support junior ones you or their mentor must observe how well they do this and give them constructive feedback about this activity. This will help to start developing the mentors of the future and is a vital part of using a peer support system.

Education support will be available from the university and is particularly important to access if you have a student who is underachieving (Watson, 2000). The education staff can also help to provide an objective person who will be able to help you with education strategies to help deal with difficult situations.

The NMC (2010a) also allows other healthcare professionals to be mentors to nursing students within their first year, as the focus of assessment is on generic skills and professional behaviour. In addition, other healthcare professionals can feed back to you on the student's receptiveness to learning from others. Structured time contributing to the care a patient receives from others will aid the student's understanding of the patient's journey and help the student to understand how effective collaboration within the healthcare team can contribute to positive patient outcomes.

Whilst support for the student is important, support for you is also important. Research has shown that mentoring can be stressful and support is necessary if mentoring is to be fully effective (Atkins and Williams, 1995). Within your team, other staff who work with your student will give you feedback on your student's performance and can help to corroborate your own observations of how your student is progressing. This can be really reassuring, especially if you have to make decisions with regard to failing a student. If others' perceptions of the student differ from your own, this can help you to reflect on why the student might perform differently with other people. Are your expectations too high or is there a clash of personalities? These issues will be explored further in Chapter 6.

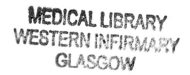
MEDICAL LIBRARY
WESTERN INFIRMARY
GLASGOW

Chapter summary

This chapter has focused on preparing to have a student and has explored the formal system of educational audit and how this can help to decide on whether the setting offers a good learning environment. Factors that contribute towards establishing a good learning environment have been discussed as well as the support mechanisms available to yourself and the student in relation to the mentor–mentee relationship.

Activities: brief outline answers

Activity 3.1 (page 33)

Your answer may include some of the following suggestions:

1. Ensuring practice learning settings provide a safe environment in which to learn:
   - health and safety induction for students;
   - moving and handling induction;
   - provision of appropriate handling equipment;
   - reporting mechanisms for accidents/untoward incidents.

2. There are appropriate learning opportunities for students within the practice learning setting:
   - orientation programme;
   - student learning pack available;
   - evidence of links between research/evidence and practice;
   - care delivery (e.g. meeting a person's hygiene needs, opportunities to practise medicine administration);
   - learning resources for students;
   - documenting care and learning opportunities.

3. There is evidence of appropriate support for students in the practice learning setting:
   - named mentor for students;
   - enough mentors to support students;
   - education support from the university;
   - preliminary, intermediate and final interviews;
   - opportunity to work with other healthcare professionals and students.

4. Students have appropriately prepared and updated mentors to provide professional support and assessment:
   - mentors are appropriately trained and updated annually;
   - students are able to work alongside their mentor;
   - staff are adequately trained to help the student learn within the specialty.

5. Care provided needs to reflect person-centred care, reflecting the rights of the clients:
   - a philosophy of care is available;
   - privacy and dignity is maintained for clients;
   - there is evidence of respect for religious and cultural needs of clients;
   - consent is sought from patients to allow students to participate in care;
   - policies and procedures are available to students;
   - effective communication is in evidence and fostered in students.

Activity 3.5 (page 38)

You may have included some of the following elements:

- organising the initial off duty to coincide with yours as far as possible;
- giving the shift patterns and hours worked;
- telling the student about their orientation programme;
- advising on how to prepare prior to the practice learning opportunity (e.g. which topics to read up on);
- finding out if the student has any specific needs or action plan they have developed;
- advising on whether catering is available in your setting or if there is a tea/coffee fund;
- providing the student learning pack or advising the student of where they can get this from;
- showing the student around the setting;
- reminding the student to bring their Ongoing Achievement Record and any other relevant documentation provided by the university.

Activity 3.7 (page 41)

Your answers may have included some of the following:

1. Registered nurses:
   - work with the student when you are not on duty;
   - provide some feedback to the student on their performance and give feedback to you as the mentor.

2. Healthcare support workers:
   - show the student around the setting;
   - help to show junior students how to deliver essential care activities such as toileting patients, meeting hygiene needs, feeding patients.

3. Senior students:
   - show the student around the setting;
   - help to demonstrate activities associated with essential care;
   - help the junior student to reflect on their experiences;
   - share their own experiences of nursing;
   - teach the student (e.g. how to undertake observations and what they might be observing/monitoring the patient for in particular situations).

4. Education representatives:
   - spend some time with the student to help them identify clear objectives;
   - help the student to reflect on experiences;
   - help the student to produce evidence to support practice achievement;
   - provide an objective person to discuss sensitive issues with or concerns they may have;
   - provide some teaching support to assist the student's learning and understanding in the practice learning setting.

5. Other healthcare professionals (these may include personnel such as the occupational therapist, physiotherapist, medical staff, discharge coordinators):
   - give students an appreciation of other healthcare worker roles and how roles complement each other;
   - demonstrate the importance of effective communication to avoid overlap and prevent omissions in care delivery.

Further reading

NMC (2010) *Education Standards for Pre-registration Nursing Programmes.* London: Nursing and Midwifery Council.
The section about the new competencies for students is useful material as it gives the mentor guidance to help them think about what the student needs to achieve for each level in the nurse education programme.

Useful website

www.nottingham.ac.uk/practice/ (recipe for successful practice learning experiences)
Nottingham website for student support leaflet. This is a leaflet written by students for students. It gives some useful advice as to how students might get the most out of their mentors.

Chapter 4
Students at different levels in their course

NMC mentor domains and the KSF

This chapter maps to the following NMC mentor domains from the *Standards to Support Learning and Assessment in Practice* (NMC, 2008b) and the NHS Knowledge and Skills Framework.

NMC mentor domains

1. Establishing effective working relationships
Demonstrate effective relationship building skills to support learning, as part of a wider inter-professional team, for a range of students in both theory and academic learning environments.

2. Facilitation of learning
Facilitate learning for a range of students, within a particular area of practice where appropriate, encouraging self-management of learning opportunities and providing support to maximise individual potential.

5. Creating an environment for learning
Create an environment for learning where practice is valued and developed that provides appropriate professional and inter-professional learning opportunities and support for learning to maximise achievement for individuals.

NHS Knowledge and Skills Framework
- Communication level 4
- Personal and people development level 4
- Health, safety and security level 3
- Quality level 2
- Learning and development level 3

> ### Chapter aims
>
> By the end of this chapter you will be able to:
>
> * explain the process of facilitating learning for your student;
> * describe how the student's Ongoing Achievement Record can help you identify how the student is progressing;
> * appreciate the importance of helping students adjust to becoming part of the nursing team;
> * describe how you can facilitate learning for a junior, intermediate and senior student.

Introduction

Whilst mentors do teach students, the main role of the mentor is to facilitate student learning and assess student competence. This chapter will focus on how to facilitate learning by helping the student move from being totally dependent to becoming an independent learner. It will also explore how you can develop students from learning essential care in Year 1, towards managing themselves and their own time with regard to care delivery in Year 2. In the third year your role is to help the student to learn how to manage a group of patients, manage other members of the team and assist in teaching colleagues.

The first step in this process is to engage students in learning how to become a nurse.

Engaging students in learning

Engaging students with regard to nursing is an important activity for you as a mentor. You need to engage students by making them welcome, feel part of the team, and by giving the students responsibilities commensurate with the level they are at on their nursing course. In doing this you will help to create a sense of responsibility in your student and will motivate the student, helping them to learn and gain the most from their practice experience.

Helping students to gain the most out of their practice requires you as a mentor to plan and facilitate student learning.

Facilitation of learning

Facilitation of learning is a complex task for the mentor to achieve, especially when time is limited and you as a mentor have many demands on your time. Your student is only one of those demands. However, it is worth spending some time to think about your student, the level they are at and what the best strategy would be to ensure their learning and development is facilitated appropriately. Facilitation is a complex skill to define, and facilitation of your student's learning will change depending on where they are at on their course.

Concept summary: Facilitation of learning

Getting Evidence into Practice: The Role and Function of Facilitation (Harvey et al., 2002)

This summary will focus on the practice development aspect of this paper. Although the paper explores facilitation in relation to getting evidence into practice, the facilitation aspects are really useful for mentors to consider. The literature review highlights key elements of facilitation and different approaches to facilitation, emphasising that the facilitator role is about supporting people to change their practice.

The findings from this literature review focus around:

- what facilitation means;
- the purpose of facilitation;
- the roles, skills and attributes of the facilitator.

The authors describe how facilitation is about enabling others, with the purpose of facilitation varying from providing help and support to achieve a specific goal, to enabling others to analyse, reflect and change their attitudes, behaviour and ways of working.

The role of facilitation involves differing approaches and can focus on 'doing'. The 'doing' role is likely to be practical and focus on support for taking on tasks. In contrast, the enabling role in facilitation is developmental in nature, seeking to help to develop an individual's potential. The enabler helps someone to learn from practice through critical reflection and dialogue between the learner and the experienced practitioner. There is a need when using facilitation to incorporate both elements.

In terms of the skills and attributes of a facilitator, this review demonstrates that any facilitator will need good interpersonal and communication skills but that other attributes may vary depending on the purpose of the facilitation. In terms of practice development they identify from a variety of authors that other attributes include being flexible, pragmatic, a risk-taker, patient, belief in the worth and value of others, as well as having the ability to create an environment of high support and high challenge.

Whilst this article reviews facilitation from a broad perspective there are key elements that are applicable to how you function with your students in practice at all levels. For a student on their first practice learning opportunity, the focus may be around the 'doing' aspect of facilitation with a move through to more of an emphasis on enabling with more senior students, once they have acquired a repertoire of skills. However, you should encourage even first-time students to begin to use reflection, helping them to become more critical as they acquire some nursing experience. As such, your dialogue with students about what they have experienced, how they can apply their theoretical knowledge to situations and how they might act differently in the future will help your student to develop into a knowledgeable doer and an able decision-maker.

The question, however, for most mentors is how do I know where to start with my student so that I can help the student to get the most out of their practice experience? The student's Ongoing Achievement Record can help you to answer this question.

The Ongoing Achievement Record (OAR)

Since the introduction by the NMC of the OAR in 2007, as a mentor you are now able to review what a student has achieved according to previous mentors. The student's strengths should be much clearer, as well as issues which have been raised with the student, action plans developed to address learning needs, and to what extent the student has achieved positive outcomes from their action plans.

The OAR is the key document in detailing a student's progress and so it is vital for you as a mentor to review this document either before or at the preliminary interview with your student.

Activity 4.1: Reflection and decision-making

Think about the purpose of the OAR. What sort of details would you wish to check in this document that would give you a sense of how your student performs in clinical practice?

A sample answer can be found at the end of this chapter.

Completing Activity 4.1 will provide you with a clear idea of what you wish to learn from the student's OAR and your list will help you to focus on your reading of a student's previous practice learning experience. However, the OAR document varies between universities and may be structured quite differently.

Activity 4.2: Critical thinking

Ask your practice education representative or the course leader on your mentor preparation programme if you can have access to a copy of the student OAR.

Using the list you completed for Activity 4.1, does the OAR provide you with the information you need to answer the key points on your list from this activity?

If you do not get a sense of your student's progress from the OAR and get answers to your key points, what do you think you could do about this?

There is no sample answer at the end of the chapter.

The OAR differs from one university to another in how it is constructed and the detail it contains. As a mentor, you can help to influence developments locally by talking to your local education representative from the university. Whilst it is true that the university will not be able to incorporate every suggestion from individuals, the universities do work in partnership with practice and should be responsive to suggestions that you have as a mentor that will aid you in developing your students. It is important to give constructive feedback regarding the OAR development if it is not meeting your needs as a mentor. Likewise, it is important for you to give positive feedback that the information in the OAR is meeting your needs as a mentor in providing you with a useful document that details your student's progress.

Setting junior students on a pathway for effective learning

When you have a first practice learning student there will be no previous input from mentors in the OAR. How you set the scene for a first year student's learning is vital in terms of preparing your student as to how they will learn effectively in a practice learning setting. This needs to be discussed early to establish what your student can expect to be learning.

Throughout the first year of a nursing programme, the NMC (2010a) states that first year students need to focus on achieving competencies that relate to essential care for patients, safety issues, professional values and how to behave as a nurse. These key areas should guide you as a mentor in what you need the student to focus on.

When your student arrives in your setting they should have developed an action plan/learning contract of what they hope to achieve and, if they visit your area prior to commencing the practice learning, it is useful to advise them to develop an action plan/learning contract before they actually start. An action plan/learning contract helps you to identify what the student's expectations are and gives you an ideal basis from which to clarify with the student what they are actually there to achieve. Action plans/learning contracts can be used as the focus for the preliminary interview and allow you as their mentor to be clear about your expectations of your student.

For many students on their first practice learning opportunity, this will be their first experience of working as part of the healthcare team, if not their first experience of being at work, and as such can be a stressful time for them.

> ### Case study: Carla, a student in her first practice learning opportunity
>
> *I felt really bad the other day, ended up crying and wondering if I could stay the course in nursing. I had been asked to do the patient's observations in one of the bays. Felt okay about this as I had taken patient's observations before. I thought I had done a good job but sister called me over to a patient and asked me why I hadn't scored this patient's Early Warning Score and reported it to my mentor.*
>
> *I had taken the patient's temperature, pulse, blood pressure, respirations and oxygen saturation level. I tried to explain I didn't know how to calculate the Early Warning Score (EWS) using the observation chart. I didn't realise it was important to calculate the score and thought I would ask my mentor about it when she had some time later. I tried to explain this to sister but she said that this patient's pulse had become really fast and irregular and the doctor needed to know about this urgently and that every patient needed this score doing when the observations had been recorded.*
>
> *When she realised I didn't know how to calculate the scores for a patient she became really cross with my mentor and said she would have words with my mentor later.*
>
> *I felt really awful – I was in trouble and it sounded like my mentor might be too. I didn't know what to do. Sister rushed away to call the doctor and I didn't know whether to tell my mentor what had happened or not.*

This case study demonstrates the importance of working alongside your junior students to ensure that they know the correct procedures they need to follow and how to recognise when a patient's condition is changing so they can alert the relevant people. First year students require a good deal of support and teaching and this takes a lot of planning. It can be really easy to forget and allocate them jobs to do without checking that they not only feel competent but are also competent to carry out your instructions. The delay in informing the doctor about the change in this patient's condition is not the student's fault. The mentor is at fault for assuming the student would be able to complete this task. However, the mentor not only put the patient (and working relationships) at risk but also increased the student's stress levels, and this may affect the student's self-esteem and confidence in their abilities in the future. The clinical environment is impossible to control and it can be hard for students to pick up what is essential (Papp et al., 2003) unless as a mentor you are directly working alongside your student, pointing out what they should be noting and learning.

The socialisation process – adjusting to being a student nurse

The first practice learning opportunity can be a critical time for student nurses and you need to try to ensure that you make the student's first experiences in healthcare positive ones.

Attrition on nursing programmes is often highest in the first practice learning opportunity and, whilst some of this may be attributed to an individual realising they have chosen the wrong profession, there is evidence that some of this may be due to initial practice learning experiences being distressing due to the sheer pace and intensity of practice learning experience, leaving students disillusioned with nursing as a career (Gibbons et al., 2007).

Healthcare teams have their own particular structure and culture and the student will need some guidance about how they fit in to your healthcare team and what they can and cannot do. It is also important to make sure that your student is supervised and their learning is planned (Papp et al., 2003) as, for many learners, their experience is that they can spend the majority of their time working alone or with other learners (Marriott, 1991) and this lack of support is a contributory factor in student attrition (Brodie et al., 2004). Working alone may ultimately increase a student's confidence, but this is not the case during a first practice learning experience. Similarly, if you ask other learners to work alongside your student you need to ensure that the learner you ask to supervise a junior student has some experience and is sufficiently competent to supervise your junior student.

Activity 4.3: Decision-making

Give some thought to your team, and who make up the individual members of the team. Who might be able to assist you in helping a first year student settle into your team?

A sample answer can be found at the end of this chapter.

As a registered nurse and mentor, students can often feel in awe of you even if you think you are a really approachable person. It is vital that the student settles into the practice learning environment and feels comfortable as, if they don't, it will impede their ability to learn. Using others such as healthcare assistants or more senior students to help the student settle in often enables them to ask questions that they may not want to bother you with as they can see you are busy or they might feel they'll appear a bit silly.

It is so easy for you to forget how intimidating the practice learning environment, patients and the staff can seem when you walk into your first practice learning opportunity, and using systems to minimise your student's fears is paramount if you want them to learn.

Focusing on essential care, patient safety, professional values and behaving as a professional

These elements are the focus of what a student needs to learn in Year 1. As a mentor you need to identify what these terms mean for you within your setting, and these will vary slightly depending on your field of nursing. You need to decide as a nursing team the benchmarks that you will utilise in order to be able to say that the student is competent. Once you have identified the elements that will enable the student to demonstrate their competence in these areas you need to decide how you will plan the student's experience so that they can achieve competence and confidence in each element. Just asking the student to follow you and observe what you do will provide them with experience but it does not mean that they will actually learn anything. Student learning needs to be a planned experience.

Activity 4.4: Reflection and decision-making

Reflect on the experiences your setting offers that will enable the student to demonstrate competence in:

- essential care;
- patient safety;
- professional values;
- behaviour as a nurse.

Identify what you would expect your student to demonstrate confidence and competence in by the end of the practice learning opportunity.

You may find it useful to agree this list with your fellow mentors.

There is no sample answer at the end of the chapter.

Having a list which clearly identifies what the student needs to achieve will ensure that you and your student remain focused on what they must achieve by the end of Year 1. This doesn't mean that your student won't be able to learn additional things but it will help to identify the minimum required for competence and will lend some consistency between mentors during the process of assessing students (this will be dealt with in more detail in Chapter 5).

Second year students

Case study: An extract from a student's learning journal

I started on this placement a week ago and am really enjoying being in this environment. I like this sort of work – it is a residential setting for individuals with complex learning needs. Some of the service users have a lot of physical disability, as well as learning difficulties. Am a bit worried though as I haven't had much experience in looking after physical problems – hope they [the staff] don't expect too much of me! My mentor said that I could take a key role in looking after one of the service users once I have settled in and got to know the routine. I want to do this but please don't let them just drop me in it! I know I've only got 18 months to go before I qualify but they will need to tell me exactly what they expect of me and show me how to do it. I just wish I'd spent more time on things like catheter care, hygiene needs and feeding people before. I wish I'd put this in my action plan. Wonder if it is too late to say I am still a bit worried about giving physical care. Perhaps I should try and get some agency work on adult wards – it'll help with my overdraft and with what I need to learn.

By the time you have a student in their second year they should be proficient in essential care skills and have acquired some basic knowledge about nursing care. However, it is important to check the student's previous performance in their OAR so that you have a sense of how the student has progressed over their first year and the type of experiences they have already had. The student should also have completed their action plan for their experience with you but it is worth discussing the action plan and how it relates to the type of experience you are offering and what you expect from the student. The student may also be afraid, as the case study highlights, to tell you how limited their experience is.

The second year in nursing can be a difficult one for students. The initial excitement of being successful in getting a place on the course can start to wear away and sometimes students experience a 'second year slump'. They are no longer very junior students and they are not yet senior students and they may feel at this point that there is a very long way to go before they finish the course or that they haven't progressed as far as they should have.

Pearcey and Elliot (2004) also identified the potential for a growing lack of motivation in student nurses as they progress on their course, which was directly linked to the student's practice learning opportunity experiences. They also highlight the impact of a positive experience on the student's motivation and how you as a mentor influence the student's impressions and experience of nursing. There is a need for you as a mentor to act as a positive role model for your student, taking care to ensure they are not out of their depth, as it is important to sustain the student's motivation and aspirations to good practice to help maintain their motivation to become a nurse (Spouse, 2000).

Stress can also build up for nursing students at this stage; they have more complex academic workloads, financial pressures may become more of a problem, as a setting you are expecting the student to take on more responsibility, and the emotional cost of nursing starts to build up (Evans and Kelly, 2004). Whilst some stress is motivating, too much stress can interfere with learning, and the support and understanding you offer students as a mentor is vital as you help the student move from delivering essential care to being able to think more critically about nursing (Field, 2004).

Activity 4.5: Decision-making

How do you think the experience you provide for a second year student should differ from that of a first year student? How will you start to plan their learning?

A sample answer can be found at the end of this chapter.

By the end of your practice learning experience the student should have become more independent in their nursing practice. This will then start to set the scene for what they will need to achieve by the end of their programme.

Third year students

Case study: An extract from the student's learning journal

I had a fantastic day today. Am exhausted trying to remember everything but feel important as part of the team for the first time. My mentor allowed me to take charge of the bay we were in. She was there to support me but expected me to plan and organise everything for the six patients we were looking after. I've come home feeling really good about myself as I managed nearly everything without my mentor having to take over. I discharged two patients, admitted three, made a referral to social services and gave handover to the physios and OT. I did feel awful when a patient fell in the toilet but I knew what to do – I did a first aid check and, as the lady seemed okay, we got her into bed and called the doctor. I even remembered to do a full set of observations to make sure she was okay and rang her daughter to inform her of what happened after the doctor had checked her over and made sure she was alright. The one thing I forgot to do was document all this in the lady's nursing notes. My mentor had to remind me about this but she said I had coped really well with a busy shift and she was really pleased with how I am getting the hang of learning to manage. I've got a great mentor as she didn't make a big thing of me forgetting the documentation. She's really good at standing back and letting me get on with things but I still feel I can ask her stuff – she doesn't make me feel like an idiot for forgetting something.

Building on what your student has achieved in Year 2, your senior student needs to develop the skills required to register as a nurse. They will still need you as a knowledgeable practitioner to support and guide them (Spouse, 2001) but at the same time you need to allow the student the right level of freedom to develop their expertise without compromising patient care. The senior student should now begin to appreciate the complexity of giving quality care and what they now require are opportunities to refine their skills in terms of managing care.

Activity 4.6: Reflection

Reflect on the nursing expertise you expect a senior student to demonstrate in order to become eligible to enter the profession as a registered nurse.

A sample answer can be found at the end of this chapter.

Your student should have an action plan/learning contract that should reflect the skills you have identified. As a mentor, it is also vital that you read the student's OAR to identify your student's previous achievement and if there are any areas that require further development before you move on to enabling the student to achieve the managerial skills you now need to focus on. Time spent discussing your expectations and how you intend to help the student to achieve the skills required is vital during the early phase of the practice learning experience.

It is also important to work directly alongside your student initially, even in their final practice learning opportunity. This gives you a sense of how confident and able the student has become and will probably only be necessary for a short period of time at this stage. Once you are satisfied that your student has settled into your setting, and that their care standards are safe, you can then begin to delegate more responsibility to them by reducing your level of supervision. You can start to allocate them a small group of patients that will allow your student to practise their managerial skills and develop their decision-making skills (Aston et al., 2010). However, it is still vital that you oversee your student's work and are there to provide a sounding board for the decisions your student makes about care delivery and how they intend to plan and organise their day.

Constant, constructive feedback to your student is vital so they are aware of how they are progressing and what aspects of their performance need to be refined further. This, together with tips on how to refine performance, can help your student to maintain their motivation (Spouse, 2000) and will help them to feel valued as a team member as they improve their performance. As your student gains confidence in their own performance, they can then start to support and teach other students.

Supporting other students

Supporting and teaching others is an integral part of the nurse's role (NMC, 2010a) and your senior students need to begin to develop this aspect of their performance.

A peer support initiative: an evaluation summary

Supervising and Supporting Student Nurses in Clinical Placements: The Peer Support Initiative (Aston and Molassiotis, 2003)

This report evaluates the allocation of junior students to a senior student for the purpose of support and teaching under the supervision of a mentor. The aim of this approach is to increase the professional responsibility of senior students through a support and teaching of clinical skills role for junior students.

continued overleaf...

continued...

The report explains how students are formally prepared for this role within the university setting and how mentors are prepared by the clinical support teacher.

Evaluation of the initiative highlights how much this type of support is appreciated by junior students, who appreciate being able to discuss their experience of the practice learning opportunity with someone who understood how they were feeling, and who made them feel at ease. In addition, help in developing essential care skills from someone who had the time to do this helped the junior student to gain in confidence in terms of their skills acquisition.

For senior students, the initiative made them examine their own nursing practice and knowledge, helped them become more organised, and highlighted how much skill and knowledge they had acquired during their education. This enhanced the senior students' confidence as nurses, helped to motivate them and assisted their own personal and professional development, especially when they received positive feedback from their mentor.

Activity 4.7: Reflection

Reflect on how you might think about developing your senior student's support and teaching abilities within your area. How might you begin to utilise the strategies you identify?

There is no sample answer at the end of this chapter.

Developing your student's confidence and competence in nursing and teaching is a complex task and requires significant input from you as the student's mentor. It is not the easy option but will help you to ensure that your students feel valued as individuals, as well as important members of your team.

Chapter summary

This chapter has explored learning in the context of you being a facilitator of learning and the support you need to provide students with in order to sustain their motivation.

It has also signposted how you might approach facilitating learning for different levels of students, utilising existing resources to enhance the student's learning. Each student you have may be quite different and the importance of the **OAR** document has been highlighted to ensure that your student's learning is facilitated from their starting point rather than working with all students in the same way.

Activities: brief outline answers

Activity 4.1 (page 49)

Your answer may include the following:

- Whether the student has achieved all previous competencies.
- What the student's timekeeping is like.
- Is there detail of sickness and absence that might be a concern?
- Is the student a reliable member of the nursing team?
- Is the student enthusiastic?
- Have previous mentors highlighted any issues that have hindered the student's achievement?
- Has the previous mentor highlighted what the student needs to focus on in your setting?
- Is there evidence the student has developed action plans/learning contracts for practice learning opportunities?
- Is there an indication in the previous mentor's comments that the student has fulfilled their action plan/learning contract?
- Overall, does the student seem to have been progressing as they should for the stage they should be at in their nursing programme?

Activity 4.3 (page 51)

Whilst all healthcare teams differ in how they are structured, you may have thought of the following:

- more senior students;
- healthcare support workers;
- receptionist or other administrative staff.

Activity 4.5 (page 54)

When you have a second year student in their practice learning opportunity they will have had a lot of input in terms of theoretical knowledge and will have acquired a repertoire of nursing skills and knowledge from previous practice learning. Your role as a mentor may include the following:

- Reading the student's OAR to ensure their action plan/learning contract is appropriate for your setting and to see the previous mentor's comments on the student's performance.
- The student will still need a settling-in period and you need to work with the student to make sure they have acquired essential care skills, safeguarding issues and professional behaviours required in Year 1.
- You can then begin to help the student to see how they can transfer their previous skills to your setting and to identify how their skills may need to be adapted to your service user group.
- Following discussions and working alongside the student you can then make it clear to the student how you want them to progress during this part of their course. This will help to focus your student on what they will be expected to achieve.
- Once you are satisfied that the student is able to transfer their essential care skills to your setting, you can encourage them to recognise, understand, anticipate, organise, plan and deliver the care for one or two patients. This will help to give the student the opportunity to start to manage themselves and their time effectively and will help them to start to prioritise care needs. They will probably need considerable support from you as they start to take on this responsibility.
- You can also encourage your student to begin to analyse the care they are giving by questioning them about why they make particular decisions about a person's care, encouraging them to use evidence to support their choices. This will help them to develop their critical thinking skills.

Activity 4.6 (page 55)

In facilitating your student's learning, they are now at the stage at which they need you to enable them by providing the sort of opportunities that will help them to:

- demonstrate professional behaviour including reliability and punctuality;
- demonstrate time management skills;
- safely manage care for a group of service users using prioritising and decision-making skills;
- provide a sound evidence base for their actions;
- work effectively as a team member;
- support other team members;
- manage others through effective delegation;
- teach others within the team.

Further reading

Aston, L, Wakefield, J and McGown, R (2010) *The Student Nurse Guide to Decision Making in Clinical Practice*. Milton Keynes: Open University Press.
This book contains a chapter that advises the students on how to get the most out of their mentor. It is useful to read as a mentor as it will provide you with some strategies in helping your student to get the most out of their learning experience whilst they are with you.

Aston, L and Molassiotis, A (2003) Supervising and Supporting Student Nurses in Clinical Placements: The Peer Support Initiative. *Nurse Education Today*, 23 (3): 202–10.
This article explores how senior students can help facilitate a junior student's learning in practice learning experiences. It also outlines how both senior and junior students can benefit from this process.

NMC (2010) *Education Standards for Pre-registration Nursing Students*. London: Nursing and Midwifery Council.
This is useful reading material for mentors to ensure you understand the background to changing to an all degree programme for nurse education and to help you understand the aims students need to achieve during the course of their nursing programme.

Useful websites

www.nmc-uk.org
This website has guidelines for universities in using and developing the Ongoing Achievement Record.

www.nottingham.ac.uk/nursing
This website has a mentor resource section that can be used to access material that will guide you in looking at portfolio material when assessing the student's underpinning knowledge that supports their nursing practice.

Chapter 5
Assessment of practice learning

NMC mentor domains and the KSF

This chapter maps to the following NMC mentor domains from the *Standards to Support Learning and Assessment in Practice* (NMC, 2008b) and the NHS Knowledge and Skills Framework.

NMC mentor domains

3. Assessment and accountability

Assess learning in order to make judgements related to the NMC standards of proficiency for entry to the register or for recording a qualification at a level above initial registration.

7. Evidence-based practice

Apply evidence-based practice to their own work and contribute to the further development of such a knowledge and practice evidence base.

8. Leadership

Demonstrate leadership skills for education within practice and academic settings.

NHS Knowledge and Skills Framework

- Communication level 4
- Personal and people development level 4
- Quality level 2
- Learning and development level 3
- People management level 2

Chapter aims

By the end of this chapter you will be able to:

- recognise your responsibilities as a mentor when conducting assessments of practice learning;
- implement a variety of strategies when assessing practice learning;
- demonstrate an understanding of what constitutes effective assessment of practice learning;
- recognise some of the complexities that might occur when assessing practice learning.

Introduction

> ## Case study: Helen
>
> *Helen is a nurse on the orthopaedic unit and is Suzie's allocated mentor. Suzie is coming to the end of her second year of training and needs to have achieved level three in each of her competencies to progress into her final year of training. Helen completed her mentor preparation years ago but due to all the changes in the Trust and having moved jobs herself, she has not been asked to mentor a student for over two years. Helen has attended her annual updates and feels reasonably up-to-date with the recent changes to nurse training, but is still unsure about completing Suzie's documentation. Suzie is a good student and has not given Helen any cause for concern but her final interview is due next week and Helen is a little worried about how to grade her and how much evidence she should expect or ask for. Helen is a very experienced practitioner and understands her mentoring responsibilities and wants her assessment of Suzie to be a good assessment. Helen decides to contact her education representative at the university for advice. The lecturer is very helpful and takes Helen through a few examples of the different types of evidence she might expect her student to produce for achievement of her competencies. The lecturer also advises Helen to consult her colleagues regarding Suzie's progress, to ask their opinions about how Suzie has developed during her practice learning experience.*

In Chapter 4 you explored your mentoring role in the facilitation of students' learning. This chapter will focus on your mentoring responsibilities to assess students' learning. Before exploring the specifics of assessment, it is important to acknowledge that thousands of nurses are trained each year with the vast majority meeting the required standards for registration. Programme providers continue to produce registered nurses of a very high standard. However, whilst learning in practice accounts for 50% of student nurse training and it is fairly common to hear of students failing an assignment or an examination, the infrequent number of students failing their practice learning experience remains concerning (Norman et al., 2002). This could be the result of having excellent high quality students, or because mentors are doing such an outstanding job in developing students so effectively they are all meeting the required standards. However, recent studies have concluded that one of the reasons students are not failing in practice is because their mentors are reluctant to award a fail grade (Duffy, 2004; Skingley et al., 2007).

Assessing the students' learning whilst they are with you in practice is one of the most important mentoring roles you will be performing. Assessing a student's learning provides you with the opportunity to nurture the student and develop their confidence as a practitioner. The overall aim of this chapter is to develop your assessing skills and confidence to ensure you are able to conduct effective assessments of your students. This in turn will make the role of sign-off mentors (see Chapter 8) easier.

This chapter is structured in line with Rowntree's (1987) classic framework for assessment: why assess, what to assess, how to assess, how to interpret and how to respond. These are some of the questions frequently raised by mentors. The chapter begins with an exploration of your responsibilities as a mentor when conducting assessments in practice, responsibilities to the student, the public and the sign-off mentors. This is followed by an exploration of the different aspects of practice learning that you will be assessing, the related student documentation, and the application of some of the theory that supports and explains what constitutes a fair and valid assessment of practice learning. The final section will introduce a number of strategies that you can use to ensure that you are able to give your students accurate constructive feedback and avoid giving any student the benefit of the doubt. Duffy (2004) highlighted in her study that some mentors, for a variety of reasons, will award a student a pass grade when they should have given them a lower grade, therefore giving them the benefit of the doubt.

The mentor's accountability and responsibilities to assess practice learning effectively

As a mentor you have a specific responsibility to assess the progress your student is making, to assess their competence in practice and confirm that they are capable (or not) of safe and effective practice (NMC, 2008b). In Chapter 2 it was highlighted that you will continue to develop your mentoring skills with every student you support. Your assessing skills do, however, need to be effective from your first day as a student's primary mentor. This does not mean that you need to be an expert in assessment, but that you need to have a good understanding of the assessment process, the student's documentation and some of the complexities that might be involved. New mentors do in general have some understanding of their facilitation of learning role but limited understanding about their assessment role and responsibilities. Your previously acquired skills of supporting, organising and planning will be of particular use if you are allocated a student who is underachieving. Adopting a systematic, structured approach when assessing the student will enable you to make accurate decisions as to the student's progress and their overall achievement.

In what has become a seminal piece of work, Kathleen Duffy (2004) confirmed what many mentors and teachers had previously believed: that a significant number of mentors were not failing students when they should have been, with 46% agreeing with the suggestion that students were sometimes allowed to pass without having gained sufficient competence. Whilst Duffy's study has contributed to the NMC standard to support learning and assessment in practice (NMC, 2008b), what is very concerning are the findings from a more recent study conducted by the *Nursing Times* (Gainsbury, 2010) which found that 37% of mentors had passed students, despite their concerns about the students' competence or attitude, or thinking they should be failed. So whilst the new NMC standard for mentorship (as it has become known) should steadily improve the quality mentoring practices, it is evident that mentors require support and continuing professional development to end the practice of giving students the benefit of the doubt.

Case study

Rachel, a Health Visitor, has been mentoring Tina during her eight-week community practice learning experience and this afternoon she has arranged to conduct Tina's final interview. Rachel has some concerns regarding Tina's achievement of two of the field-specific competencies. During the interview Rachel

continued overleaf...

continued...

> *gradually works through each of the competencies, looking at the evidence Tina has produced to support her achievement for the level required. After assessing all the evidence produced by Tina, Rachel still feels she has not met the minimum standard needed for level four and begins to feed this back to Tina. Tina immediately breaks down in tears, saying she knows she can do better, and that if she doesn't pass she will be thrown off the course, and nursing is all she has ever wanted to do. She has been working extra shifts as an HCA to supplement her bursary and has been very tired. Rachel gives Tina the benefit of the doubt and awards Tina a pass for all her competencies.*

Activity 5.1: Reflection

List the reasons why you feel some mentors might give students the benefit of the doubt.

A sample answer can be found at the end of this chapter.

You may have mentioned that the mentor concerned might not know how to complete the student's paperwork, or does not have the confidence in their own mentoring abilities as reasons for passing a student when they should have failed them or given them a lower grade. Duffy's findings support this view; in her study she asked: *Why are some student nurses being allowed to pass clinical assessments without having demonstrated sufficient competence?* The following four categories were developed from the data gathered.

Research summary: Reasons for failing to fail

The four categories of reasons are:

1. leaving it too late;
2. personal consequences to both the student or mentor;
3. facing personal challenges;
4. experience and confidence.

To avoid leaving the student's assessments until too late, the organisational and planning skills that you use in everyday practice can now be transferred and used in the planning of assessing the student's progress. You may have observed a colleague who has had to rush the completion of their student's paperwork on the very last day of the practice learning experience as they have not been able to find time to complete the student's final interview earlier, or in some instances taken the documentation home to complete. Whilst it is the student's responsibility to arrange the date and time for their progress interviews with their mentor, consider for a moment how you are going to guide your student to ensure the interviews happen at the appropriate times and that the final assessment is not rushed. Whilst the consequences for patients of registering students who have not met the required standards are often acknowledged, it is also worth considering the impact of failing to fail on the student concerned. How can a student improve if they are not given accurate feedback regarding their competence? A student could progress through their training unaware that they are not up to standard. Unfortunately it is sometimes the case that a student reaches their final management practice learning opportunity before they are identified as an underachieving student; this scenario then has huge consequences for the student concerned. The content of the following sections have been developed to help you to recognise and address some of the issues identified by the mentors in Duffy's work, to improve your confidence as an assessor of practice learning.

What is assessment of practice learning?

You will be very familiar with the term assessment as used in relation to the delivery of care, but what do you understand about assessment of practice learning? You may suggest that it involves some form of measurement of skills and understanding, of whether someone is competent or not. Rowntree (1987) offers a fairly comprehensive and straightforward definition of assessment by stating: *Assessment occurs whenever one person in some kind of interaction, direct or indirect, with another is conscious of obtaining and interpreting information about the knowledge and understanding or abilities and attitudes of this other person.* Apart from student nurses, do you currently assess anyone else's learning? You may have included preceptors or HCA NVQ assessments in your answer. As the nursing profession strives to work increasingly inter-professionally so the opportunities and requirements to assess your colleagues' learning also increases. Did you also include patients, carers and relatives?

From a broad perspective, assessment of learning is a generic term for a set of processes that measure the outcomes of a student's learning, which in relation to nurse training and their learning in practice are their competencies. The NMC has adopted the following definition of competence: *the combination of skills, knowledge and attitudes, values and technical abilities that underpin safe and effective nursing practice and interventions* (adapted from Queensland Nursing Council, 2009). The NMC's competency framework identifies the standard of practice that is required of your students before they can become registered practitioners. The framework contains 40 generic competencies, plus the relevant field-specific competencies (formally known as branches), of which there are 19 for adult and learning disability and 21 for mental health and child. These competencies have been grouped under four headings:

- professional values;
- communication and interpersonal skills;
- nursing practice and decision-making;
- leadership, management and team working.

As you can see from the new domains, the skills the student will have to acquire reflect the future role of the nurse. By the end of their training your student will have been assessed and hopefully met the requirements for each generic competency and those in their chosen field.

Activity 5.2: Critical thinking

Take a moment to consider what you feel are the purposes of assessing learning in practice.

A sample answer can be found at the end of this chapter.

Purpose of assessing learning in practice

In response to the previous activity you may feel that the main purpose of assessing learning in practice is to maintain high standards of patient care, or to give the student feedback on their progress. In your role of mentor you have a responsibility to assess students during their training to enable them to register as competent practitioners to protect the public (NMC, 2008b). However, the purpose of assessment is much more than the passing or failing of a student; it is very much about motivating and developing your student to deliver best practice. Meeting the NMC code of professional conduct also requires that you *manage oneself, one's practice, and that of others.* This involves the delegation of different aspects of care delivery to your colleagues, requiring some form of assessment of their abilities for safe and effective delegation. Once you have assessed your student you will know how much supervision they require and whether that is direct or indirect supervision.

Effective assessment of practice learning

You should now have a good understanding of why you are assessing practice learning and of your mentoring responsibilities relating to assessment. The next step is your development as an assessor. This involves providing you with a clear understanding of what an effective assessment is, and an opportunity to explore a range of approaches you can use to improve your effectiveness as an assessor, providing you with one piece of the jigsaw that is successful mentoring. Quinn and Hughes (2007) suggest that for any assessment to be a good assessment it needs to have validity, reliability, discriminatory powers and be practicable: these are known as the cardinal criteria for assessment.

How to strengthen the validity of your assessments

Validity, according to Quinn and Hughes (2007), is *the most important aspect of any test and is the extent to which the test measures what it is designed to measure.* For example, how valid would your assessment be if you were assessing your student's ability to give a subcutaneous injection by asking them questions about how they would perform the skill? The validity of your assessment would be stronger if you were to observe them performing the skill. Observation is by far the most valid method for assessing practice. The NMC (2008b, page 32) states that *most assessment of competence should be undertaken through direct observation in practice.* It is an NMC requirement that students are always supervised either directly or indirectly and that they have access to a mentor for a minimum 40% of their time in practice. However, this also acknowledges that it is not feasible for mentors to be able to observe every aspect of their student's practice. This is where you expect your student to gather evidence of being observed delivering practice by your colleagues; this evidence is often referred to as 'witness statements' or 'observed learning records'.

Quinn and Hughes go on to explore the concept of validity in greater depth, one aspect of which is particularly relevant to assessment of practice learning: predictive validity. Predictive validity is the extent to which an assessment is designed and delivered to predict the student's future behaviour, which is highly relevant in your assessment of a student's overall competency.

To help strengthen the validity of your assessments consider the following question and make a few notes: how can you ensure that the student you have assessed will continue to deliver care to the same standard when you are not there to observe them?

A sample answer can be found at the end of this chapter.

You may have included in your answer that you would need to observe the student's practice a number of times with a variety of patients and that this would give you confidence that their practice was consistent, strengthening the predictive validity of your assessments. This would involve you practising continuous assessment.

Continuous assessment

During your own training you will have been assessed in practice, no matter how long ago or how recently you qualified. Take a moment to remember how you were assessed during your training. You may have completed the ward-based practical assessments which consisted of one aseptic technique, one drug round, one total patient care and one ward management assessment. These types of assessment are called episodic, one-off assessments. A major drawback of this method of assessing was that it relied on the student's performance on the day of the test and therefore did not necessarily reflect how the student might perform in general over longer periods of time (Quinn and Hughes, 2007). There was much criticism of the one-off assessments and they were superseded by continuous assessment, which has since become established in many education institutions (Neary, 2000) and continues to be the chosen approach for pre-registration nurse training. There is a danger, however, that continuous assessment could become a one-off assessment if it is not implemented appropriately; this would subsequently reduce the predictive validity of those assessments.

Activity 5.4: Leadership and management

What do you understand about continuous assessment? What might be the strengths and weaknesses of you using continuous assessment? Make a few notes.

A sample answer can be found at the end of this chapter.

You may have noted that continuous assessment is an ongoing process, like taking regular snapshots of your student's practice and giving frequent feedback, a series of progressively updated measurements of a student's achievement and progress. Using a continuous approach to your assessments will ensure that you are measuring the knowledge, skills and attitudes of your student over a period of time, helping to strengthen the validity of your assessments, overcoming some of the shortcomings of episodic (one-off) assessment. For example, when taking a driving test, who would you say had a more accurate picture of your driving skills: the driving instructor or the examiner?

A continuous approach to assessment often involves both formative and summative elements, helping to give some structure to the overall process. Formative assessment refers to the feedback that you give to the student about how they are progressing at regular intervals during their practice learning experience so they can address any areas of their practice they need to develop. The intermediate interview is a formal opportunity for formative assessment. In addition to the intermediate interview, giving the student feedback on their performance on a more regular basis will make sure the student has been given every opportunity to improve, and will inform you, giving you the confidence to accurately judge their level of achievement. As the student's mentor you will also be required to conduct the student's summative assessment at the end of their practice learning experience, where you assess their level of achievement against their generic and field-specific competencies; this is the final overall judgement. Should your student have taken significant periods of sick leave during their practice learning experience, you may feel unable to complete a summative assessment of the student. This would depend on how much time off they have taken and if you feel you could make a valid assessment of their competency based on the evidence the student has produced.

In considering the strengths and weaknesses of continuous assessment, it is likely that you identified lack of time as one of its major constraints. You might also have noted that obtaining regular feedback as to how your student is progressing will make your overall judgement of their level of achievement more accurate and make you feel more able to deliver effective feedback to them. Walton and Reeves (1999) suggest that by using continuous assessment students should maintain the level of competence, and also that they will be graded to their expected level.

Where students are allocated in a traditional way, using a practice learning experience as a block of learning (e.g. eight weeks on a surgical or medical setting), adopting a continuous approach to your assessments is relatively easy. With the introduction of a 'learning pathways' (hub and spoke) approach to the allocation of students, mentors might consider this to be more challenging to continuous assessment as they will be required to assess evidence produced and verified by the mentors supporting their students during a 'spoke' practice learning experience. If your programme providers are using the 'hub and spoke' approach to practice learning, it would be useful for you to consider how you can facilitate a continuous approach to the assessment of your students.

How to strengthen the discriminatory powers of your assessments

As previously stated, one of the main purposes of assessment is to protect the public by ensuring that only those students who have met the required standard of achievement register as nurses. Your assessments therefore need to differentiate between those students who are at the required level and those students who are not. This is referred to as the discriminatory powers of assessment. Unfortunately we have all come across a practitioner about whom we wonder 'how on earth did they qualify?' Do you feel that you are effective at discriminating between different student's abilities: the student who has achieved the required level of competency and the one who has not? Can you tell the difference between the HCA who has met the criteria for NVQ level 3 and the HCA who is still at NVQ 2?

Activity 5.5: Critical thinking

Consider an aspect of patient care and ask yourself the following questions:

- How do I know if someone is competent or not at delivering this care?
- What am I looking for?

An outline answer is provided at the end of this chapter.

In looking to strengthen your powers of discrimination you may start by comparing one student with another student both at the same stage of training. This is called norm-referenced assessment. Can you see any problems with this approach? You could, for instance, have recently been allocated a number of relatively poor students; if you are comparing them against each other the standard for achievement, the norm, could be lowered and students might therefore be awarded a pass grade. However, if you had compared the said student with students who have greater abilities you might have awarded them a fail grade. If norm-referenced assessment is the main method of assessing practice learning, this could challenge the validity and reliability of those assessments and hence your effectiveness as an assessor.

Using a criterion-referenced approach to your assessments will help to strengthen the effectiveness of your assessments. Criterion-referenced assessment, as the term suggests, involves using a list of criteria against which you assess the student's progress. Over the years different schools of nursing have developed assessment documentation for the students containing specific criteria for mentors to measure their student against to see if they have met their outcomes and proficiencies. These are now known as competencies and the documentation is the Ongoing Achievement Record (OAR), which was covered earlier in Chapter 4.

The use of the term competency in the literature can be ambiguous and confusing at times (McMullan et al., 2003). In pre-registration nurse training, competency refers to the *knowledge, skills and attitudes required by the nurse at the point of registration. A competency describes the nurse's skills and abilities to practise safely and effectively without the need for direct supervision* (NMC, 2010a). To add further add clarification of the concept of competency, Short (1984) suggested that there are different approaches to continuous assessment of competency, ranging from a behavioural approach where performance is demonstrated to a more humanistic approach which uses a more holistic approach to assessment. What you are aiming to assess is the capacity of the student to integrate knowledge, values, attitudes and skills in the world of practice (Gonczi, 1994).

To strengthen the discrimination of the assessments, assessment strategies include tools that help mentors differentiate between the student's levels of performance. Steinaker and Bell (1979) identify five levels of skill acquisition that can be used when assessing practice learning: exposure, participation, identification, internalisation and dissemination. Alternatively, Bondy (1983) developed what she refers to as *criteria for clinical evaluation*, which consist of three aspects to the assessment.

> ## Theory summary: Criteria for clinical evaluation (Bondy, 1983)
>
> 1. The professional standard – the student's behaviour should be safe not only for the patient but also for her/his colleagues and others.
> 2. The quality of performance – this relates to the amount of time, equipment, space and energy a student uses when delivering an aspect of care, and how confident and relaxed they are.
> 3. The assistance required – how many cues does a student require to maintain effective performance? How closely does she/he require supervising?

An interpretation of the above criteria used locally is the degree of supervision a student requires, ranging from constant supervision graded at level 1 through to minimal supervision graded at level 4. The NMC has a requirement that there are two progression points within a student's training programme; these are usually at the end of Years 1 and 2. For practice learning, a student is required to achieve their competencies at a certain level before being allowed to progress to the next year. An exploration of your student's practice assessment documentation will clarify what is expected of your students at the progression points. Utilising a form of criteria like Bondy levels will strengthen your ability to discriminate between different students' performance at their progression points.

How to strengthen the reliability of your assessments

To increase your effectiveness as an assessor, the assessments you conduct need to have reliability. Reliability according to Quinn and Hughes (2007) is *the term used to indicate the consistency with which a test measures what it is designed to measure.* For instance, if you were having a really bad day, how would you make sure that the results of any assessments you performed that day would be the same as those you would perform if you were having a really good day? This is given the term intra-mentor reliability. Rowntree (1987) suggests that assessment can never be purely objective, that there will always be an element of subjectivity due to human involvement in the process.

Inter-mentor reliability, however, proposes many serious challenges; this relates to the consistency across mentors. Consider the mentors you work with and how likely it is that they would all come to the same conclusions if assessing the same student's competency and award the student exactly the same levels of achievement. It is possible that you will have come across students undertaking their NMC essential skill clusters (ESC) assessments. The ESC assessments apply to all students who started their training from September 2008 onwards (NMC, 2007a). The NMC introduced the ESCs to address some of the concerns about skills development that were raised in their review of fitness to practice. The aim of the ESCs is to provide clarity and increase the public and the profession's confidence in nurse training. The ESCs are generic skills statements that have been developed to complement the competencies set out in the NMC Standard (2010a) and have provided HEIs and Practice Practitioners with an opportunity to strengthen mentor reliability.

The ESC assessments may be implemented slightly differently by different universities, so it is important for you to clarify with your local HEIs how they have chosen to implement them and explore any relating documentation. Generally a one-off summative assessment method is being used, which runs in conjunction with the normal continuous assessment of competencies process. This effectively means that the student is assessed using a pass or fail system, including second attempts if required, and that they continue to show progression and development of the skills throughout their training.

Case study: Student and mentor dialogue

Tom is a second year student and his mentor Libby is preparing him for his medicine administration ESC assessment.

Libby: *OK, Tom, you have been observing me over the last few days doing the drug round for our patients, do you feel ready to start practising for your medicine essential skill cluster assessment?*

Tom: *Yes, I think so; this one really bothers me. I am sure I will get something wrong, there is so much to remember.*

Libby: *Don't worry, you will get plenty of practice. I will also arrange for you to do any injections that have been prescribed.*

Tom: *But I won't have to do them all for my assessment, will I?*

Libby: *Yes you will, the NMC says that you need to administer medicines via routes commonly used in this area.*

Tom: *Yes, but I am only a second year and will be assessed again on drug administration and injections on all my future placements.*

Libby: *Yes, but here we do quite a few subcutaneous injections so they should be part of the assessment.*

Tom: *But that isn't fair, Claire did her medicine assessment here with her mentor last week and her mentor told her she didn't need to do any injections.*

Activity 5.6: Critical thinking

Consider how you can ensure when assessing students that your expectations of the student are, as far as possible, the same as those of other mentors.

A sample answer can be found at the end of this chapter.

Your answer may have included having a clear understanding of the student's competencies and what is expected for each competency. To strengthen the reliability of your assessment you need to be aware of any factors that might bias your assessments either favourably (error of leniency) or harshly (error of severity), often referred to as the 'halo' or 'devil' effect. You might, for example, feel that you understand what is expected of the student but because you really like the student and get on well with them, you might give them a grade which is a little higher than their actual performance, and of course, alternatively, you might have a student you don't get on with and grade them slightly lower than their actual performance deserves.

At the heart of assessment is the mentor's professional judgement (McMullan et al., 2003), so to strengthen the inter-mentor reliability practitioners require the opportunity for support and continuing professional development that encourages them to reflect on their mentoring practice.

However, no assessment schedule can ever be 'assessor proof', as each assessor has their own interpretation of competence (McMullan et al., 2003).

Activity 5.7: Critical thinking

What should students be expecting of you as an assessor?

A sample answer can be found at the end of this chapter.

How to strengthen the practicability or utility of your assessments

One of your responses to the activity above might have been that you give students time to feed back on how they are progressing. Quinn and Hughes (2007) acknowledge that assessments must be practical, in that the time it takes to do the assessments, and the costs involved, are appropriate. For instance, it would be ideal if a mentor could have the same supernumerary status as the students, as this would enable them to hand over patient care to facilitate giving the student feedback on their progress, but this is not reasonable to expect.

Giving comprehensive, accurate and constructive feedback to your students is fundamental to your effectiveness as a mentor. For a student to grow and develop they need to know how much progress they are making. Towards the end of a practice learning experience both student and mentor should be coming to similar conclusions about the grades that will be awarded; there should be no surprises for the student at the final interview. Anecdotal evidence from students is often critical of mentors who give rather generalised, superficial feedback, stating that their students 'are doing well' or 'they will make a good nurse', but nothing more constructive. Through continuously assessing your student and giving them frequent constructive feedback you can play a significant role in the development of your student's confidence and help towards strengthening the practicability of your assessments so everything is not left until the last minute, when it is usually not possible to find the time needed.

Chapter summary

The overall aim of this chapter has been to develop your skills, enabling you to effectively assess practice learning. Strengthening the validity, reliability and discriminatory powers or the practicality of your assessments is a little like a balancing act. The more tools and criteria you use to increase validity, reliability and discriminatory powers, the more time-consuming and less practical your assessments can become. The purpose of examining this underpinning theory is for you to consider what you can reasonably address to avoid giving any of your students the benefit of the doubt.

Activities: brief outline answers

Activity 5.1 (page 62)

You may have included some of the following in your answer:

- the mentor is not confident enough;
- the student will improve on their next practice learning experience;
- not sure how to fail the student;
- do not want to be the one to end a student's career;
- not sure about the student's paperwork.

Activity 5.2 (page 63)

You may have included some of the following in your answer:

- to monitor the student's progress;
- to guide you as to how closely or not they need to be supervised;
- to inform the content of your feedback;
- to motivate the student;
- to give you feedback on how well you are teaching the student.

Activity 5.3 (page 65)

You may have included some of the following in your answer:

- by role-modelling your own consistently high standards of care delivery;
- by observing the student's practice on a number of occasions with different patients;
- by developing understanding in the student regarding maintaining standards of care;
- by consulting colleagues the student is working with;
- by asking the student to give you feedback regarding their practice.

Activity 5.4 (page 65)

You may have included some of the following in your answer:

- ongoing monitoring of the student's progress;
- regular assessments;
- frequent observations of the student's practice;
- getting feedback about the student from colleagues;
- completing the student's documents throughout the practice learning experience, not just at the end of it.

Strengths of using continuous assessment:

- real-world assessment;
- obtain an overall picture of the student's abilities;
- opportunity for continually updating and setting goals;
- opportunity to give frequent feedback;
- opportunity to develop the student's reflection skills;
- opportunity to develop the student's problem-solving skills;
- helps to more accurately measure competence and future behaviour;
- student should know how well they are performing; therefore, no surprises at the end of the assessment period.

Problems of using continuous assessment:

- time-consuming;
- continuous pressure on the student;
- may be influenced by bias;
- difficult to coordinate shift working.

Activity 5.5 (page 67)

You may have included some of the following in your answer:

- they communicate well with the patient;
- they deliver the care effectively;
- they can evidence base their practice;
- they understand the rationale for the care;
- they know their own limitations;
- they can recognise any potential problems and know who to report them to.

Activity 5.6 (page 69)

You may have included some of the following in your answer:

- by assessing the student against the competencies in the booklets;
- by keeping yourself up-to-date of changes to the students training;
- by discussing the competencies with other mentors;
- by having a good understanding of the different levels of achievement and what is expected at each level.

Activity 5.7 (page 70)

You may have included some of the following in your answer:

- they knew what you expected from them;
- you put them at ease;
- they trust you to give you honest constructive feedback;
- you are knowledgeable and use evidence based practice;
- that you gave them time to prepare for the assessment;
- that the assessment took place during a less busy time on the ward.

Further reading

Walton, J and Reeves, M (1999) *Assessment of Clinical Practice: The Why, Who, When and How of Assessing Nursing Practice*. Wiltshire: Cromwell Press.
This text is particularly helpful in developing a clear understanding of how the principles of assessment of practice learning can be applied to practice.

Sharples, K et al. (2007) Supporting Mentors in Practice. *Nursing Standard*, 22 (39): 44–7.
This paper outlines useful guidance for mentors when supporting underachieving students.

Useful website

www.nmc-uk.org
By accessing this website mentors can keep up-to-date with NMC directed curriculum changes.

Chapter 6
The challenging student

> **NMC mentor domains and the KSF**
>
> This chapter maps to the following NMC mentor domains from the *Standards to Support Learning and Assessment in Practice* (NMC, 2008b) and the NHS Knowledge and Skills Framework.
>
> **NMC mentor domains**
>
> **1. Establishing effective working relationships**
> Demonstrate effective relationship building skills to support learning, as part of a wider inter-professional team, for a range of students in both theory and academic learning environments.
>
> **2. Facilitation of learning**
> Facilitate learning for a range of students, within a particular area of practice where appropriate, encouraging self-management of learning opportunities and providing support to maximise individual potential.
>
> **3. Assessment and accountability**
> Assess learning in order to make judgements related to the NMC standards of proficiency for entry to the register or for recording a qualification at a level above initial registration.
>
> **4. Evaluation of learning**
> Determine strategies for evaluating learning in practice and academic settings to ensure that the NMC standards of proficiency for registration or recording a qualification at a level above initial registration have been met.
>
> **5. Creating an environment for learning**
> Create an environment for learning where practice is valued and developed that provides appropriate professional and inter-professional learning opportunities and support for learning to maximise achievement for individuals.
>
> **6. Context of practice**
> Support learning within a context of practice that reflects healthcare and educational policies, managing change to ensure that particular professional needs are met within a learning environment that also supports practice development.

continued overleaf...

continued...

8. Leadership

Demonstrate leadership skills for education within practice and academic settings.

NHS Knowledge and Skills Framework

- Communication level 4
- Personal and people development level 4
- Health, safety and security level 3
- Service improvement level 2
- Quality level 2
- Learning and development level 3

Chapter aims

By the end of this chapter you will be able to:

- identify the components that help you to decide competence;
- describe what is meant by a challenging student;
- explore why a student may be challenging;
- explain strategies that can be utilised when dealing with a challenging student;
- ascertain the support mechanisms available to you when dealing with challenging students;
- utilise strategies in dealing with failing students;
- construct and use action plans to help the student towards achievement;
- recognise your own needs as a mentor.

Introduction

All students need to be assessed during their time in your practice learning area (see Chapter 5), with the mentoring process helping you to determine what level of competence the student has achieved by the end of their practice learning experience. When you have a student who seems to fit in with the team and performs well in terms of their own and your expected development, mentoring is a relatively easy process compared with having students who present as a challenge to you for whatever reason. Determining the student's competence, though, is not an easy process.

Activity 6.1: Critical thinking

Kate is a second year student. She works really hard and is keen to develop her nursing skills. Kate has observed her mentor undertaking urinary catheterisation on several female patients and is keen to 'have a go' herself.

An elderly lady needs intermittent catheterisation performed on a regular basis. Kate explains why she needs to do the procedure and the potential problems that can occur. She also shows her mentor through direct observation that she can prepare the equipment safely, undertake the procedure according to the local policy, measure and record the amount of urine drained, dispose of the used equipment, and effectively clean the trolley she has used.

If you were her mentor, would you say that Kate is competent in undertaking this procedure?

A sample answer can be found at the end of this chapter.

Defining competence

The NMC (2002) uses the term competence to describe the skills and ability to practice safely and effectively without the need for being supervised directly. In Kate's example, if you use the NMC definition of competence, Kate cannot be competent as defined by the NMC as she needed her mentor to directly observe her undertaking this procedure. So, although Kate performed the procedure correctly, she still needs to practise this skill before she can be deemed competent in it. However, competence is what the NMC requires your student to achieve by the end of their programme of study. This is why most universities use frameworks to indicate where the student should be by a specific point in the course. This helps to guide you in your judgement of each student and you should always refer to whichever framework your school of nursing is using to determine whether the student is progressing as they should.

Cowan et al. (2007) present a detailed literature review of various definitions of competence in nursing practice, highlighting that there is little consensus on the definition of competence with regard to nursing practice. What emerges from this literature review is a holistic notion of competence where you as a mentor need to assess the capacity of your student to integrate knowledge, skills, values and attitudes into their practice (Gonczi, 1994) with your student also demonstrating that they can transfer their learning into different contexts (McMullen et al., 2003). It tends to be relatively easy to assess someone's ability to undertake a specific skill but much harder to assess the art of nursing and human aspects of nursing such as empathy, attentive listening and appropriate responses to situations your student has to deal with (McAllister, 1998).

Within nursing, most students are able to achieve competence in its holistic sense but some students have a great deal of difficulty in developing competence, presenting challenges to you as a mentor.

Why is your student challenging?

Activity 6.2: Reflection

Think about the challenging students that either you or other mentors have worked with. In terms of nursing performance, which sort of elements made you think of the student as a challenge to you/the mentor?

A sample answer can be found at the end of this chapter.

A challenging student can be defined as someone you find difficult to deal with or someone who is not fulfilling your expectations of what they should be achieving at a particular point in their course.

The first thing you will need to undertake is a root cause analysis by reflecting on why your student might appear to be challenging. This process will involve talking to your student, reading through their Ongoing Achievement Record to try to identify trends, and reflecting on whether you as a mentor might be a cause for the student's challenging behaviour and/or low performance.

Activity 6.3: Critical thinking

Think about why a student might present as a challenging student and make a note of your thoughts.

Useful tip: It will be helpful to you to consider both causes that may lie with the student or yourself as a mentor.

A sample answer can be found at the end of this chapter.

Root cause analysis can be a complex activity to undertake. When you meet individuals, your first impressions can have a powerful effect on how you perceive them. Rather than assume that the student's performance is their fault you will need to consider all of the factors identified in your list of why a student might be challenging. Finding out why your student is challenging will help you to assist the student in developing an appropriate action plan or course of action.

It is also important, as a mentor, to take your pastoral role seriously, demonstrating that you care about the student and considering how you can help to build a student's confidence (Gunner, 1988). This will include getting to know the student to try to identify what is causing them problems with functioning in a positive way as a student.

Case study: Reflection in practice

Patricia is an experienced mentor

I had two second year students in the same group on the ward and I was mentoring both of them. Sally was really enthusiastic and got stuck in straight away and really seemed to be enjoying the placement whilst Joy didn't seem to be performing very well. She seemed very slow and reluctant to take on responsibilities. I started to think, 'I'm sure we've got a problem here'.

I sat and thought about it at home. Joy seemed a nice girl, but nice isn't enough. I asked both Sally and Joy to write a reflective account of what they had learned on the following shift and, when reading them, realised Joy might be a reflector. I then reflected on what had been written and thought about what I'd learned about learning styles on my mentor course. I realised that Sally was obviously an activist and welcomed new challenges but Joy did appear to be a reflector. I started to use a different approach with Joy. I gave her time and plenty of opportunity to discuss things with me so she had a chance to think things through before she took on new responsibilities.

It really paid off after a couple of weeks. Joy really blossomed and became a really good member of the team. It made me think about how easily I could have labelled Joy as lazy and lacking in initiative. I was so glad I remembered about learning styles and how they can affect how someone acts.

(For further information about learning styles see Honey and Mumford (1992).)

This mentor obviously thought long and hard about why this student didn't appear to be performing as well as the other student from the same student cohort. The student's experience could have been affected throughout her practice learning opportunity as could the summative assessment that the mentor undertakes on a student. It is always important to reflect on why your student may not be performing well, and to consider the problem from a variety of angles.

Stress and anxiety

Stress and anxiety are often key factors when a student is not performing well. A major source of stress comes from a lack of professional knowledge and skills, particularly for junior students (Sheu et al., 2002). For students with some experience, it may be that previous mentors have failed the student by not being good role models or through failing to address issues by guiding the student and developing action plans to give the student a constructive way forward in developing their clinical practice. As a mentor you need to provide the student with constructive and timely feedback which focuses on your student's development and not just on their deficiencies as a student (Hart and Rotem, 1994).

Case study

Gemma is mentor to Sadie, a second year student nurse who has been on her current practice learning opportunity for four weeks.

Gemma: *Sadie, I am really worried about your progress on this placement. You are really kind and caring to your patients but I expect you at this stage in your course to be using a little more*

continued overleaf...

continued... ••

> *initiative. I am continually having to ask you to do routine tasks that I actually expect a first year student to know about. I am going to give you two patients tomorrow and I expect you to think about the care you are giving, prioritise these patients' needs, deliver that care and feed back to me on your progress.*
>
> At this point, Sadie bursts into tears.
>
> Sadie: *I know I'm rubbish, it's all too much for me! I try to do things right but am so scared of doing the wrong thing. You all seem so busy that I don't like to pester you. Oh, God, I am never going to make it!*

Activity 6.4: Reflection

Take some time to reflect on this situation. What was positive about this interaction and how might the situation have been handled in a more positive way?

A sample answer can be found at the end of this chapter.

Whilst you may not consider yourself an authority figure who might be a bit scary to a student, Higgins and McCarthy (2005) found in their research that students often did not approach staff for help because they were scared of being refused help or of being annoying. They also found that if a mentor had confidence in the student, the student was more willing to assume responsibility and become independent.

In Sadie's case, it appears that lack of supervision and approachability of previous mentors contributed to Sadie's predicament. Although it is not the mentor's fault, it is evident that they are going to have to supervise and guide Sadie for a period of time to build up her confidence before they can make a judgement about her competence. It may also be the case that Sadie has not experienced that type of setting before. She may have been out in the community working under direct supervision all of the time or in a different area such as a clinic where the routine was quite different to experience in her present practice learning opportunity.

It is, however, always useful to clearly document issues as they arise, your expected behaviours by the student, how the student is going to achieve the desired behaviour, and the time by which you expect the student's performance to improve. The sample action plan in Figure 6.1 might give you some ideas of how to construct your agreed plan of action with the student.

This action plan clearly specifies what you want the student to achieve. It also demonstrates that you expect them to ask questions and check things out with you. The clearer you are with your documentation, the less room there is for misinterpretation of what you expect from the student. You will also need to remember to ensure that both you and the student sign and date all documentation so that the student cannot claim that you didn't involve them in the process or inform them of what you intend to do. The framework your school of nursing uses to guide you will also help you to articulate exactly what the student needs to be achieving.

Date	Action	Review date	Signature
18.06.11	1. Sadie will work alongside me for the next week to observe how I manage and organise my time. 2. We will set aside ten minutes at the end of the shift to discuss how the day went and to allow time for any questions Sadie has with regard to nursing care, decisions made and how I managed my time. 3. After one week, I will allocate Sadie to two patients under less direct supervision so that she can plan and organise the care effectively for these two patients. Sadie will also need to refer back to myself to discuss her plans at the beginning of the shift and we will evaluate her performance at the end of each shift.	27.06.11	Liz Aston

Figure 6.1: Sample action plan

Expectations of the student's performance

Thinking about your expectations of a student's performance and discussing these expectations within your team will help to give some consistency within your setting with regard to planning the experience and assessing your students. This can help to prevent you having too high or too low an expectation of your student's performance. It is often also helpful to write these down as a guide for all mentors and to ensure some consistency between mentors. Doing this will also assist the student to appreciate exactly what they need to do.

Case study: Reflection

First year student: Lucy

It's really good on this placement. Before I started, they gave me a student learning pack when I went to get my off duty and say hello to the staff. I read it through and it made it really clear what I needed to do to get myself ready for starting there and what would be expected of me in order to pass my competencies. I wish I'd had it on my first placement – things would have been so much easier.

Lucy highlights the importance of setting out clear expectations for your students. It also helps her to have the right level of expectation for herself and should help to prevent her trying to act outside of what is required and her level of competence. If you don't already have a student pack, you would find it useful to develop one for your practice setting. If you do already have a learning pack, it might be useful to review it to make sure it helps the student to understand the sort of performance you expect from students at particular stages in their programme. This can be especially important for the student who is a little unsure of themselves.

Self-esteem and motivation to learn

Resilient individuals who have a high self-esteem view difficult tasks as challenges to be overcome instead of problems to be avoided (McLaughlin et al., 2008). Individuals with low self-esteem can present as challenging students who appear to have a low level of motivation to learn. If your student is not coping effectively in practice learning, the problem can manifest as social symptoms where they don't interact with others effectively, emotional symptoms or physical symptoms (Sheu et al., 2002). In not coping effectively, your student may appear uninterested and avoid engaging with activities and patients in your setting. This can lead you to label the student lazy, strange or rude and can be a really difficult situation to deal with.

Start by talking to your student. It may just be that your student needs to build their confidence up a little within a supportive environment. If you take an interest in your student, make them feel that they have something to contribute, and give them support and permission to seek advice from you. This can start to build up their confidence. Providing a supportive and caring environment can have a really positive effect on your student's performance and can be really rewarding for you as their mentor as they become more confident in their professional role.

However, your student may have personal problems that are affecting the way they view themselves, or their confidence when facing new challenges. They might also have discovered that nursing is not what they thought it would be but lack the confidence to go and talk to someone about it. It could also be a more significant problem for the individual that originates from their prior experience in life. No-one is expecting you as a mentor to deal with these issues alone as they often require a lot of time and the student may need expert support.

Activity 6.5: Team working

Find out about the support mechanisms that are available to the student from their local university.

You may find it useful to chat to your link lecturer/practice learning support lecturer, who will be able to provide you with information you can pass on to your student.

There is no sample answer at the end of this chapter.

Dealing with enquiring students

It is not always the student who is lacking in confidence that can be challenging. You may have a really interested student who is very bright but is challenging because they ask questions all the time, sometimes at inappropriate times. These students can be quite difficult to deal with as you don't want to squash their enthusiasm for learning but it can be quite draining on you as a mentor and can have an impact on your patients.

Case study

Rebecca is a first year student who, prior to starting her nursing course, has undertaken a degree in biology. She is a really enthusiastic student, who makes it very clear she wants to learn as much as possible. Whilst you are helping Rebecca to wash a patient who is terminally ill and in a rather drowsy state, Rebecca starts to ask you about what sort of changes she needs to look for in the patient to help her to recognise this patient's end is near. This makes you really angry as you are concerned the patient will be aware of what Rebecca is asking.

Activity 6.6: Critical thinking

How might you deal with this type of situation?

A sample answer can be found at the end of this chapter.

The enquiring student can be just as challenging as the student who lacks motivation, and may need help to redirect their energies and enthusiasm without dampening down their enthusiasm for learning and making them afraid of asking questions. You may need them to appreciate that there are times when it is not appropriate to ask questions and that they need to have some insight into how you as their mentor may be feeling.

However, not all students are relatively easy to deal with. There may be situations where you try several different strategies with your student and still feel you are not improving the situation.

Dealing with failing students

You have identified the problem with your student's performance, developed an action plan with clear timescales, and the situation has still not improved. If the student still has time within the setting you will need to re-think your action plan. Everything will need to be documented, either in the Ongoing Achievement Record or, if space doesn't allow for this, on separate sheets of paper which can be dated, signed and forwarded to the student's personal tutor. At this stage it will also be useful, if you haven't already done so, to involve the link lecturer/lecturer support person for your setting or the student's personal tutor.

If the student is at the end of their practice learning with you, this stage will form the summative assessment for the student. It may be useful to check with your peer mentors and/or manager as well as with other healthcare professionals the student has worked with, before you undertake the assessment to ascertain their view of your student's performance. This can help to reassure you that your judgement matches with their views, or can help to reduce any personal biases you may have with regard to the student.

> ## Case study: Karen's reflections
>
> *I had a third year student who didn't seem to be functioning at the right level for where she was on the course. Over a few shifts it became apparent that she wasn't even functioning in the way that I would expect someone who was at the end of their first year. After talking to her and developing an action plan that wasn't achieved, I spoke to the link teacher and my manager. The link teacher and I saw the student together and talked through the issues, tried to find out if there was anything outside of work that was affecting her, and developed a new action plan. The guidance from the link teacher was really useful but still didn't work. I even got my student to work with other staff in case it was me that was having this effect on her. It came to the end of the student's placement and I realised that this student wouldn't achieve quite a lot of her competencies and that I would have to fail her on some of the competencies. I was really nervous about doing this as I had always managed to turn situations around successfully before. The link teacher asked me if I wanted her present for the final interview. I said I wanted to do this by myself but wanted her support to be available if I needed her. The link teacher reassured me that she would be in her office if I should need her.*
>
> *The interview with the student was difficult but I managed to do it by myself and document everything.*
>
> *It really upset me as I felt I had failed my student. My manager and the link teacher listened to my worries and helped to support me through this. Although I hope I don't get this situation again, I feel a little bit more confident that I could deal with it.*

Failing students is never a very easy task but, with the right support, it can be managed with minimal trauma to both the mentor and the student. It is important to access the support that is available for both yourself and the student. Mentors often blame themselves feeling that they should be able to facilitate achievement for students and, on rare occasions, this is just not possible. What is important is that you satisfy yourself that you have been objective and have facilitated opportunities to give your student a chance to achieve requirements in your setting.

Second attempts at practice

For students who fail to achieve at their first attempts at practice competencies, universities will have different examination regulations. You will need to check with your partner university as to how many further attempts are allowed. All universities will make provision for students to have at least one further attempt at gaining practice competencies.

Activity 6.7: Communication

What do you think your responsibilities as a mentor are when explaining to your student why they have failed to achieve their competencies?

A sample answer can be found at the end of this chapter.

These situations are difficult for you as a mentor, for the practice learning setting as a whole and for your student, particularly if this is your student's final attempt at gaining their required competencies. It would be most unusual for your student not to be upset in a situation such as this. However, it is unfair to both your student and members of the public to avoid giving this feedback. The public have a right to be cared for by individuals who have demonstrated the competencies required by the NMC to an appropriate level in order to progress towards the level required for entry to the profession. Your student has a right to be given honest feedback without being given the benefit of the doubt (Duffy, 2004) as their expectations about what is required of them need to be realistic. Ultimately, the sign-off mentor needs evidence of any particular trends that have been identified with your student in order for them to make an appropriate judgement that enables the student to gain entry to the nursing register. It is important for you to recognise that the student may have the right of appeal to a committee within the university if this is their final attempt at achieving their practice competencies.

Appeal systems for students

Universities have in place appeal systems for students if there are extenuating circumstances that may have affected their performance in the practice learning setting. These systems are in place to ensure that the student is able to disclose any information alongside evidence to support their claim. The committee may decide that the circumstances have contributed to the student's poor performance. The end result of an appeal may mean that your student has an attempt at gaining competence voided, thus giving them another attempt to gain competence. Conversely, it may be that the committee doesn't feel the extenuating circumstances have hindered the student's performance and the student may have their course discontinued.

Looking after yourself as a mentor

When you have a challenging student and manage to turn the situation around for a student and they succeed it can be extremely rewarding – a job well done. However, it can be really stressful and upsetting for you when this doesn't happen. Facing situations with challenging students who don't seem to respond, or be able to respond, to your support and constructive advice can make you feel you have failed them as a mentor. It can also be time-consuming and can affect the ward morale as a whole.

It is useful to reflect on your experiences to try to ascertain if there was anything else you could have done and, if possible, learn from this for the future. Reflection can also be reassuring as you begin to realise you did the best you could, given the time and resources available to you. You need to realise that your student has to take responsibility for their own performance, or lack of it.

Sometimes it is reassuring when you identify from the Ongoing Achievement Record that this is a trend that previous mentors have also tried to address. Occasionally, there is no previous record and this can occur for two reasons. Firstly, it may be that previous mentors have avoided addressing difficult issues. Secondly, it may just be that a student is fine when they are being told what to do all the time but they just can't seem to make the transition to acting without direct supervision. However difficult these situations are you need to always remember that if you give the benefit of the doubt to your student you could be putting patients at risk in the future.

Getting support for yourself

You need to remember that there is support you can access. Support systems vary depending on local systems that are in place but should always include:

- other mentors that you work with;
- your setting manager;
- link lecturers/practice learning support lecturer;
- the student's personal tutor.

If you are faced with a challenging student it is always useful to seek support early on. You don't need to handle these sorts of situations by yourself. Pick someone you feel comfortable talking to and whom you respect so you feel more confident seeking their help.

Chapter summary

Throughout this chapter you have explored how difficult it can be to define what competence actually means. This was followed by exploring what is meant by a challenging student and the need to explore the root cause of the issues you identify. The importance of accurate record-keeping was also emphasised as well as the need to be very specific when highlighting issues with students. The chapter briefly touched on how dealing with challenging students can affect you as a mentor as well as the support mechanisms you can use to help you through challenging situations.

Activities: brief outline answers

Activity 6.1 (page 75)

In terms of thinking about preparing for a procedure, documentation and disposal of equipment, Kate has, on this occasion, demonstrated her competence in performing a specific skill. She has also demonstrated her knowledge of why this lady needed intermittent catheterisation and the potential effects this procedure can have on an individual. However, you need to think back to what you have learned in Chapter 5. Assessing students requires you to assess knowledge, skills, values and attitudes. There is no evidence in the account presented of how Kate approached and reassured this person, or whether she protected the patient's privacy and dignity whilst performing this skill.

In addition, although Kate has demonstrated some competence in undertaking the procedure for this lady, continuous assessment requires you to observe behaviours consistently before you can say they have achieved competence in a particular skill.

Activity 6.2 (page 76)

You may have thought of some of the following issues:

- lacking in clinical skills;
- slow to learn and adapt nursing skills to new situations;
- poor professional attributes;
- failure to recognise limitations;
- persistent inappropriate challenging of the mentor;
- poor team-working skills;
- lack of interest and motivation;
- unreliable and lacks punctuality.

Activity 6.3 (page 76)

Mentor issues may include the following:

- Are your expectations of the student too high?
- The student may have lacked good role models in where they worked before.
- Failure by previous mentors in that they have not spent time guiding the student and developing action plans to work towards helping them to succeed.

Student issues may include:

- anxiety;
- personal problems;
- type of previous experience;
- expectations – are the student's expectations of themselves too low or too high?;
- wrong career choice;
- is the student not appreciating that they are acting outside of their limitations as a student?;
- learning style.

Activity 6.4 (page 78)

Gemma has identified Sadie's positive attributes, which is reassuring for the student. However, she does this after she has already said that she is really concerned about Sadie's progress. Sadie was probably still assimilating the comment that her mentor is concerned and probably won't have registered the positive comment about her.

In terms of the action plan identified, this may well have the effect of setting the student up to fail even if this is not the intention. It might have been better to have asked Sadie to work with her (Gemma) for a few days to observe how she organises her work, encouraging her to ask questions about how Gemma organises her work. Taking a few minutes to reflect together (maybe at coffee time) to explore what went well on the shift in relation to how and why Gemma made specific decisions would have been a valuable learning opportunity for Sadie. When her confidence had improved, Gemma could then have allocated Sadie two patients to take responsibility for, reassuring her that it is okay to check out the decisions she is thinking of making to make sure they are safe and effective decisions. In doing this, it shows Sadie she is allowed to ask questions and approach Gemma with issues. It can be important for students to know that they have to do this.

Activity 6.6 (page 81)

You may have thought of the following:

- Ask Rebecca to leave any questions until later.
- Demonstrate that the patient may well be aware of her surroundings by talking through what you are doing and asking permission to wash parts of her.
- Talk to Rebecca after you have completed the procedure, explaining that you understand she may not have known but that even patients who are in a coma may still retain their hearing and awareness of what is happening around them.

- Ask Rebecca to make a mental note of any questions and to keep a small notebook in her pocket to jot questions down in so she can ask you at a time when you can give her your full attention.
- Ask Rebecca to undertake some reading around the subject of caring for the terminally ill patient and communication issues so she can increase her knowledge and do some reflective writing on her experience with this patient.
- Review Rebecca's findings from her reading and her reflection so you can ensure that she is learning from her experience and now appreciates that some of her questions may well distress patients.
- If Rebecca has found some interesting articles, praise her for this and say what you may have learned from her search of the literature and how much you appreciate her providing you with some new material for reflection.

Activity 6.7 (page 82)

You may have included some of the following:

- Ensure you have privacy and enough time to talk through issues with your student.
- Be supportive – your student will probably be very distressed.
- Emphasise your student's strengths and good qualities.
- Be very clear about exactly what your student has not achieved and how you have reached this conclusion.
- Give specific advice about what your student needs to do in order to improve their performance.
- Document everything you have discussed – don't forget to include the date, time and the signatures of everyone present.
- If you have not already done so, inform your student's personal tutor and/or the link lecturer/ practice learning support person.

Further reading

Duffy, K (2004) *Failing Students: A Qualitative Study of Factors that Influence the Decisions Regarding Assessment of Students' Competence in Practice.* Glasgow: Caledonian University.
Duffy's work is a seminal piece of research that explores why mentors may fail to fail students. It gives some insight into the emotional component of dealing with students who may not be achieving well and how this can affect both the student and mentor.

Useful website

www.nottingham.ac.uk/practice
The mentor resource part of this website is a useful section to 'dip into' to help you develop your mentoring skills.

Chapter 7
Disability issues

NMC mentor domains and the KSF

This chapter maps to the following NMC mentor domains from the *Standards to Support Learning and Assessment in Practice* (NMC, 2008b) and the NHS Knowledge and Skills Framework.

NMC mentor domains

1. Establishing effective working relationships
Demonstrate effective relationship building skills to support learning, as part of a wider inter-professional team, for a range of students in both theory and academic learning environments.

2. Facilitation of learning
Facilitate learning for a range of students, within a particular area of practice where appropriate, encouraging self-management of learning opportunities and providing support to maximise individual potential.

3. Assessment and accountability
Assess learning in order to make judgements related to the NMC standards of proficiency for entry to the register or for recording a qualification at a level above initial registration.

5. Creating an environment for learning
Create an environment for learning where practice is valued and developed that provides appropriate professional and inter-professional learning opportunities and support for learning to maximise achievement for individuals.

6. Context of practice
Support learning within a context of practice that reflects healthcare and educational policies, managing change to ensure that particular professional needs are met within a learning environment that also supports practice development.

8. Leadership
Demonstrate leadership skills for education within practice and academic settings.

continued overleaf...

continued...

NHS Knowledge and Skills Framework
- Communication level 4
- Personal and people development level 4
- Health, safety and security level 3
- Service improvement level 2
- Quality level 2
- Equality and diversity level 3
- Learning and development level 3

Chapter aims

By the end of this chapter you will be able to:
- define what is meant by disability;
- explore your role in preventing discrimination;
- understand your role and responsibilities in mentoring a student with a disability;
- explore what is meant by reasonable adjustments for someone with a disability;
- explore measures to assist you in enabling your student to achieve.

Introduction

Case study

Clare is a second year adult branch student who has ME. Most of the time Clare is able to prevent a relapse by making sure she doesn't get overtired. Your setting operates a 12-hour shift pattern and the ward manager likes to ensure that all students work the same pattern of off duty as their allocated mentor. Clare has a letter from the Occupational Health Department stating that she is only able to work six hours per day. This makes it difficult for you as you work a 12-hour shift pattern, which means that Clare will have to work some shifts without your support.

Activity 7.1: Decision-making

Think about how you would deal with this situation.
- Do you feel it is acceptable to make special arrangements for your student?
- How could you ensure that Clare has support and supervision when you are not on duty?

A sample answer can be found at the end of this chapter.

The number of disabled students (including those with dyslexia) has increased over the last ten years (Ijiri and Kudzma, 2000; Hoong Sim and Fong, 2008), and it is required by law that both educational and practice settings make reasonable adjustments for students (Equality Act, 2010). Whilst the law states that reasonable adjustments must be made, it is less clear what is a reasonable adjustment to make. This can sometimes make it difficult for you to make decisions about how to facilitate learning for someone with a **disability**. In addition, it is often the negative aspects of a disability that are identified whereas there can be positive aspects to the disabilities people have. For example, heightened empathy, innovative flair, lateral thinking and problem-solving skills are traits shared by many dyslexic individuals (Morris and Turnbull, 2007), and these are very useful traits to possess in nursing. This chapter endeavours to explore some examples of the types of situations you might encounter when mentoring students. A useful starting point is to consider what is meant by disability.

Defining disability

Activity 7.2: Reflection

Reflect on your understanding of what disability means and identify the categories of disability you might come across when mentoring students.

A sample answer can be found at the end of this chapter.

Konur (2002) highlights that it is important to think about access to nurse education for disabled students and the subsequent service provision these students will need, highlighting that nursing programmes cannot deny admission to applicants based on their disability. What can present problems though is the issue of 'fitness to practice': this is a requirement for nursing, but the judgement of what is meant by fitness to practice has been left as a local issue to interpret (Morris and Turnbull, 2006). In addition, the NMC (2004b) requires evidence of good health and character, with the NMC stating that the concept of good health is a relative concept. This can make it difficult for education institutions, service provider organisations and mentors to make clear judgements about a student's fitness to continue on a nursing programme at times. This can be a particular concern for mentors who feel vulnerable sometimes when making decisions. You are not expected to be an expert in disability issues: the university staff that you liaise with will be able to help you with any concerns and how you might overcome these concerns as they will have disability liaison officers who are experienced in giving guidance on disability issues. However, students do not necessarily have to inform you if they have a disability.

Confidentiality issues

All students coming into nursing have occupational health screening to see if they are fit to undertake nursing programmes. If individuals are accepted onto a nursing programme after occupational health screening, they are not required to disclose their disability to education or practice staff (Sanderson-Mann and McCandless, 2005). If the student chooses not to disclose personal information to you as their mentor, you cannot be expected to make reasonable adjustments for them.

If the student does tell you that they have a disability, confidentiality is a key issue in terms of knowledge about the student's disability. Students, in general, report a reluctance to disclose information about their disabilities (Blankfield, 2001) as they worry about discrimination in terms of job opportunities once they qualify, as well as being labelled and stigmatised whilst undertaking the course (Barga, 1996).

Case study

Gemma is a third year student nurse on practice learning opportunity who is dyslexic.

I really worry about my dyslexia, particularly when I start a new placement, as I don't function too well when I am anxious and unsure of things. I try to take my time to organise myself by making detailed notes so I don't forget anything, particularly as I am expected to manage a small group of patients now. I like to re-check everything I have written down and take some time to think about what I need to do first and what I can ask other people to do for me. I haven't told anyone apart from Alice my mentor about my dyslexia as I don't like people to think I am thick. People sometimes do think that. My mentor seemed really nice and supportive, that's why I told her about my dyslexia.

Yesterday, though, I overheard one of the other staff nurses moaning about me being too slow to function properly in this area. My mentor told her not to judge me too harshly as I had dyslexia. I was mortified! I didn't want everyone to know.

Activity 7.3: Reflection

Do you think Alice was right to tell the other staff nurse about Gemma's dyslexia?

Could there have been another way to handle the comments from the other staff nurse?

A sample answer can be found at the end of this chapter.

One of Gemma's concerns was about being labelled and possibly discriminated against, which is against the law – you need to take steps to prevent discrimination in your sphere of practice.

Preventing discrimination

Despite numerous anti-discriminatory campaigns there tends to be assumptions and concerns about the employability of disabled people in the UK, particularly within health-related professions (DOH 2000), although there is little evidence to support these assumptions and concerns.

Activity 7.4: Reflection

Think about the organisation you work in: how many disabled nurses are you aware of? Are you aware of any support systems that your organisation has in place for someone with a disability?

There is no sample answer at the end of this chapter.

Your reflection on Activity 8.4 will depend on the environment you work in and your own experience of working alongside someone with a disability. Of course, you may be unaware of individuals who have a disability as many individuals with a disability try to hide their disabilities to prevent them from being seen as different. Individuals use strategies to conceal their disability through a fear of being misjudged or experiencing rejection, ridicule and stigmatisation (Barga, 1996; Illingworth, 2005).

The Equality Act (2010) makes it illegal to discriminate against a person with a disability, with discrimination being defined as a person being treated unfavourably because of something connected with their disability and the unfavourable treatment cannot be justified.

Case study

Jane is a third year student who has dyslexia and, in particular, has been having some difficulty in reading and interpreting prescription charts when helping on the medicines round.

Jane disclosed her dyslexia to her mentor and she has received a lot of help and support from both her mentor and her university to help her to manage in clinical practice learning opportunities. Jane needs to complete her Essential Skills Cluster assessment in medicines administration before the end of this practice learning opportunity, which is in one week's time. Jane's university rules are that there are only two formal attempts at this assessment. Jane feels ready to take this assessment, but her mentor is concerned that she will not pass the assessment as she is still having difficulty in reading and interpreting the prescription charts accurately.

All of Jane's peers have already passed this assessment and she feels she should be allowed to do it and to have some allowance made for her disability. Her mentor explains that she can't make allowances for Jane because, in order to complete the course successfully, the student needs to demonstrate that they are safe in administering medicines under supervision. Jane's mentor suggests contacting the university to get some more advice and support on how to proceed and to seek help to assist Jane towards achievement, but Jane is insistent she wants to go ahead and says she feels discriminated against because of her disclosing her disability.

Activity 7.5: Critical thinking

Do you think Jane is being discriminated against? Consider the case study carefully in order to provide rationales for your answer.

A sample answer can be found at the end of this chapter.

Accusations of discrimination can be very difficult to deal with and can be distressing for the mentor, the setting team and for the student. The answer is to try to prevent such accusations by working towards supporting your student, and seeking specialist advice about support for your student and the sort of coping strategies that could help your student to achieve. It is also worth checking the student's Ongoing Achievement Record to see if other mentors have identified problems in the student achieving previously, and what sort of methods they have used to assist the student in developing their competence in whatever aspect they are finding difficult. Making reasonable adjustments for students does not mean making it easier to help your student achieve by reducing the standards required in order to function effectively within the profession.

Case study

Alex is a first year mature student who has a health problem which affects his stamina and ability to complete a full shift without periods of rest. He manages activities without difficulty but does get very tired at times and needs to take a few minutes' rest on a regular basis during his shifts at work. Alex brought a letter from his personal tutor about needing frequent breaks. His mentor talked to Alex about this on his first day and he explained he could manage but just needed permission to have a ten-minute break every two to three hours. Alex's mentor stated this was not possible as it is a very busy area and the break times are set to cover the area adequately as patients need to know nurses can respond to their needs promptly. The mentor also said that it wouldn't be fair to other staff and that it might affect how he was able to achieve his competencies.

Activity 7.6: Decision-making

Think about how you might handle such a situation. Is it reasonable to refuse this request? Would this request affect Alex's abilities to achieve his competencies?

A sample answer can be found at the end of this chapter.

This case study highlights a reasonable adjustment that can be made to accommodate disability. As long as Alex achieves the competencies required in this practice learning opportunity, there is no stipulation that Alex has to work exactly the same shifts as other members of staff. You need to be supportive and flexible to help your students get the most out of your setting and achieve the required competencies.

It might be argued by some mentors that Alex won't be able to take frequent breaks when he is a qualified nurse. This argument does not stand up to scrutiny as Alex may, after discussion with his employer, have his needs accommodated by his employer. Part of the issue here is what is considered a reasonable adjustment by employers, and what the organisation can do in terms of reasonable adjustment. It is unfortunate that there is not more specific guidance for employers on specific issues as disability can be highly variable in how it affects an individual. These issues are left to individual employers although an employer will have to be able to justify the decision that they make. Employers cannot discriminate on the grounds of disability alone. Alternatively, Alex might choose to undertake part-time work, or he may take full-time employment where his job is less physically demanding.

Helping students with a disability to have a successful practice learning opportunity

As discussed in Chapter 3, the approachability of you as a mentor is crucial when dealing with your student, and is particularly important when you have a student who has a disability. Morris and Turnbull (2007) found in their research that the student's perception of their mentor's personal qualities was a major factor when considering whether to tell their mentor if they have a disability. They also found that the length of practice learning opportunities was a significant factor influencing disclosure of a disability and propose that this might be due to the opportunity to develop a trusting relationship with the mentor. Whilst you cannot immediately influence the length of a student's practice learning opportunity, you can influence how easily your student might confide in you. By being welcoming and taking an interest in your student as a person from your first meeting, a good rapport can usually be easily established. First impressions can be really influential in establishing a good relationship, but can also be difficult to rectify if you appear rushed and dismissive of the student at your first meeting.

Activity 7.7: Reflection

Think about how you might conduct your first meeting with your student. How might you try to establish a supportive relationship from this initial meeting?

A sample answer can be found at the end of this chapter.

Stress and anxiety can affect anyone's performance, and having a disability may well add to the usual stress that most students experience when starting a new practice learning opportunity. By being a mentor who is ready to provide effective support for all students, this can help when you have a student who is uncertain of whether to tell someone whether they have a disability. By being approachable to your students, this can help to make them feel safe in terms of disclosing personal information to you that might impact on how they perform in clinical practice.

Coping strategies that students might find helpful

In Activity 8.6, we explored Alex's specific needs around frequent rests, which is a coping strategy that works for Alex whilst still enabling him to be successful on his nursing programme.

Sometimes coping strategies can be easy to identify and accommodate. At other times, coping strategies might require some practice from the student and significant support from the mentor to achieve, which can be difficult in a busy environment, but not impossible. Students with dyslexia, for instance, may use a variety of resources and/or strategies to ensure their patients' safety. Some individuals with dyslexia use hyper-vigilance and constant re-checking of things to try to ensure they don't miss or forget anything. They may need to make handwritten or computerised lists to help them function effectively. According to Bartlett and Moody (2001), these types of strategy are not surprising when difficulties in processing information are a key feature in a dyslexic adult. However, coping strategies that may work for one individual may not be successful with another individual who has a similar disability.

Activity 7.8: Decision-making

Imagine your student has told you that they have a disability and that they need extra help from you because of some problem in achieving competencies in a previous practice learning opportunity. If you had no idea how to help the student, who might you seek help and support from?

A sample answer can be found at the end of this chapter.

As a mentor you can't be expected to be an expert in all aspects of disability and the coping strategies that might be useful. It is really important to seek expert help and be supportive of the student with regard to the coping strategies that might be suggested by others, as long as it is reasonable to do so. Suggested strategies might be very easy to implement such as allowing your student extra time to complete tasks or organise themselves in preparation for what you need the student to do. This requires some thought from you as a mentor in terms of planning the student's experience in order to enable them to have the best chance of being successful.

Documenting action plans

Obviously it will be important to document the action plans you develop for your student in the student's practice assessment record. Documentation varies across universities but most documentation of relevant action plans is included in the student's Ongoing Achievement Record. However, do take care when documenting issues relating to the student's disability as you will need the student's permission to include mention of their disability as all other mentors will be able to access this record of achievement. It should only be necessary to document what your student's progress is or any difficulties they are having in achieving the required competencies.

Students who fail to achieve competence

Providing students with a supportive environment, and supporting your student with suggested coping strategies, does not necessarily mean that they will achieve all of their competencies to the required level. What you need to do as a mentor though is to ensure you have taken every opportunity to facilitate learning opportunities that might help your student to achieve, document these, and ensure both you and the student sign them. This helps to prevent misunderstandings and assures all relevant parties that you have discussed any issues with your student. Your clear documentation will also help to provide an audit trail of the measures used to support the student, specific action plans, and outcomes from action plans.

It can be traumatic and stressful for both the student and you as a mentor when you are concerned about a student's performance and you may need to fail them in some competencies as was discussed in Chapter 6. As a mentor you may feel even more concerned when you are aware that the student has a disability. Your responsibility as a mentor is to ensure that you can justify your decision based on fact and not on any preconceived ideas about disabled individuals and their ability to attain competence (Hoong Sin and Fong, 2008).

Chapter summary

Within this chapter you have explored what is meant by disability, and how you as a mentor can help to prevent discrimination by being supportive of the student and endeavouring to provide the student with the best possible chance of achieving competence. You have also explored your role in helping to make reasonable adjustments for your student in order to help them be successful in your area and, where the student has not achieved what can be reasonably expected of a student, the need to document action plans and outcomes to provide an audit trail of the measures you have used to help facilitate your student's learning.

Activities: brief outline answers

Activity 7.1 (page 88)

The law states that where a disability is concerned you must make reasonable adjustments (Equality Act, 2010). It is obviously felt that Clare is able to cope with the demands of her nursing programme and she has managed to complete the first year of her programme successfully. It is reasonable to enable Clare to complete her chosen course by allowing her to take longer to complete the practice component of the programme due to her working six-hour shifts. However, as you cannot change your working pattern so that she has support and supervision most of the time, you will need to make arrangements for supervision for Clare when you are not on duty. It would be useful to plan her rota so she works with you as much as possible, ensuring that you make arrangements for when you are not present. If there isn't another qualified mentor available when you are not present, it is perfectly acceptable for you to arrange Clare to work under the supervision of a registered nurse who has not yet completed mentorship training. It is good practice to make sure that Clare knows who will supervise her when you are not present, and for you to communicate regularly with Clare's other supervisors to ensure that they are aware of Clare's learning needs and to check on her progress. You do need to ensure that Clare is supervised by a mentor at least 40% of her time in your setting (NMC, 2008b).

Activity 7.2 (page 89)

You may have considered the following examples:

- physical disability such as asthma, chronic fatigue syndrome, speech disability, hearing loss, loss of a limb, partial sight;
- learning disability such as dyslexia, dyscaculia, reading difficulty;
- mental health problems such as depression, schizophrenia, anxiety, personality disorders.

Activity 7.3 (page 90)

Alice was obviously concerned that Gemma shouldn't be labelled slow and unable to cope and was probably trying to protect Gemma. However, Alice did break Gemma's trust. Whilst Gemma may not have specifically said she didn't want anyone else to know, it seems unreasonable to break that person's confidence when there wasn't an overriding reason such as a compromise to patient safety. There is some evidence that mentors do have overtly critical attitudes to individuals with dyslexia (Morris and Turnbull, 2007) and by telling others about Gemma's disability, Alice may inadvertently be contributing to other staff becoming critical of Gemma's performance.

In terms of dealing with the situation in another way, it might have been more appropriate for Alice to have reminded the other staff nurse that Gemma is still a student and getting to grips with the setting routine, as well as the type of patients she is looking after, so she is bound to be slower than one of the trained staff. In addition, she could have explained how well Gemma was doing, the progress she was making and how she felt more comfortable about a student who was careful and planned things in detail than someone who might miss key things by rushing in without a clear plan of action.

You may have thought of other solutions to Alice's dilemma but breaking the student's confidence is not the answer and it could have repercussions for Alice should Gemma make a formal complaint about this incident. However well intentioned Alice's action was it is worth remembering as a mentor that you need the student's permission to share personal information about a student.

Activity 7.5 (page 92)

You may have considered some of the following issues:

It is reasonable to expect Jane to pass this assessment without allowances being made for her disability as it is an NMC requirement. However, she does need help and support with this particular issue and her mentor is right to suggest seeking more advice and support from the experts in this field as there may be other coping strategies that could help Jane to be successful. The NMC requires this particular competency to be achieved and, as a registered nurse, she will be required to be able to function without direct supervision from others.

If the mentor had not been supportive and had not suggested seeking some further help, then it could possibly be discrimination. It is important for you as a mentor to be supportive towards students, and try different strategies to help your student succeed, but it is also important to satisfy yourself as a mentor that the student will be able to function as a registered nurse.

Activity 7.6 (page 92)

It would seem unreasonable to refuse such a request. Alex is a student and is therefore supernumerary and should not be counted in the numbers of staff required to care for your group of patients. Alex is also able to undertake the same activities that other staff have to undertake and so it shouldn't affect his ability to achieve his competencies in your setting.

What it will require is some planning and support from you as his mentor to ensure that he manages to get these brief periods of rest. You may have thought about leaving this with Alex to let you know when he needs to disappear from the ward for a few minutes.

It would also seem reasonable for you to obtain Alex's permission to let the other staff know about his needs for when you might not be working alongside him. This would help to prevent any difficult situations for Alex should other staff feel resentful of these short breaks because they aren't aware of his needs.

If you are concerned that Alex might not be completing the required number of hours in your setting, you could talk this through with Alex and his personal tutor or the disability liaison person in the university to clarify the situation.

Activity 7.7 (page 93)

Your answer may have included the following:

- Being friendly at the first meeting; demonstrating that the student is expected.
- You may wish to ask all students if there is anything you can do to help them settle in quickly and you might ask them if they have any particular requirements whilst they are with you. Asking the student if they have any specific needs may actually give them the opportunity to explain what their disability is and what sort of coping strategies they have developed to help them succeed.

By asking questions such as these, it can help to prevent a lot of stress for your student and anxiety they may feel about approaching you for any specific help.

Activity 7.8 (page 94)

You would need to explain to your student that you need to get some help with the best way to help them and, with the permission of the student, you may have thought of approaching the following people:

- your peers or your manager;
- the link teacher for your practice learning opportunity setting;
- the student's personal tutor;
- the disability liaison officer for the university.

Further reading

Equality Act (2010) *Equality Act 2010: What do I Need to Know? Disability Quick Start Guide.* London: Government Equalities Office.
This publication gives in-depth information on disability with some examples to highlight the points included in the Act.

NMC (2010) *Requirements for Good Health and Good Character*, Guidance 06/04. London: Nursing and Midwifery Council.
This publication contains vital information for all mentors, especially sign-off mentors in relation to good health and character.

Sanderson-Mann, J and McCandless, F (2005) Guidelines to the United Kingdom Disability Discrimination Act (DDA) 1995 and the Special Educational Needs and Disability Act (SENDA) 2001 with Regard to Nurse Education and Dyslexia. *Nurse Education Today,* 25 (7): 542–9.
This is a very useful summary that provides a simple but useful guide to a very complex issue.

Useful websites

Rcn.org.uk/support/diversity/useful_links/disability_issues
This website contains a wealth of relevant information about disability issues in nursing and can be used as a resource to look up specific issues relating to disability.

www.nmc-uk.org
This website has the current guidelines in relation to disability issues for students in the practice setting.

www.nottingham.ac.uk/academicsupport
This website has guidance to students on disability issues in nursing.

www.direct.gov.uk/en/DisabledPeople
See this website for all the current policies in relation to employment and disability issues.

Chapter 8
The sign-off mentor role

NMC mentor domains and the KSF

This chapter maps to the following NMC mentor domains from the *Standards to Support Learning and Assessment in Practice* (NMC, 2008b) and the NHS Knowledge and Skills Framework.

NMC mentor domains

1. Establishing effective working relationships
Demonstrate effective relationship building skills to support learning, as part of a wider inter-professional team, for a range of students in both theory and academic learning environments.

2. Facilitation of learning
Facilitate learning for a range of students, within a particular area of practice where appropriate, encouraging self-management of learning opportunities and providing support to maximise individual potential.

3. Assessment and accountability
Assess learning in order to make judgements related to the NMC standards of proficiency for entry to the register or for recording a qualification at a level above initial registration.

5. Creating an environment for learning
Create an environment for learning where practice is valued and developed that provides appropriate professional and inter-professional learning opportunities and support for learning to maximise achievement for individuals.

6. Context of practice
Support learning within a context of practice that reflects healthcare and educational policies, managing change to ensure that particular professional needs are met within a learning environment that also supports practice development.

8. Leadership
Demonstrate leadership skills for education within practice and academic settings.

continued overleaf...

continued...

NHS Knowledge and Skills Framework
- Communication level 4
- Personal and people development level 4
- Health, safety and security level 3
- Quality level 2
- Learning and development level 3

Chapter aims

By the end of this chapter you will be able to:

- explain the importance of the sign-off mentor role;
- outline the criteria that need to be achieved to become a sign-off mentor;
- describe how all mentors contribute to the sign-off process;
- explain how to become a sign-off mentor;
- describe how to support other mentors to achieve sign-off status.

Introduction: What is a sign-off mentor?

Case study

Jane is a senior staff nurse who is the education representative for her practice learning opportunity setting. She has responsibility for allocating students to an appropriate mentor. She has three management students coming next month but only has one other sign-off mentor in her setting apart from herself. Although Jane is aware that a single mentor can supervise up to three students at a time, she likes to allocate one student to a mentor if she possibly can. She does have a mentor, Sally, whom she feels is ready to take on sign-off mentor responsibilities and wonders if she can get her ready for this role by next month.

Activity 8.1: Decision-making

Find out your local processes for becoming a sign-off mentor. Will it be possible to help Sally to become a sign-off mentor before next month using your local processes?

There is no sample answer at the end of the chapter.

In response to concerns about the consistency of assessment of students and the potential for unsuitable individuals to enter the nursing and midwifery professions, the NMC identified an enhanced final practice learning opportunity mentor role with additional responsibilities: the sign-off mentor role (Andrews et al., 2010). This sign-off mentor role is a new arrangement and is required for all pre-registration nursing and midwifery students who started their programme on or after September 2007. This means that this role has only been operationalised recently, so there is little literature yet available about the challenges that the role might engender.

A sign-off mentor is an experienced mentor who has completed an NMC-approved mentor preparation programme, fulfilled additional criteria and received supervision in signing off management students before being able to sign off competencies for a student in their final management practice learning opportunity on their pre-registration programme (NMC, 2008b). For midwifery students, all mentors who have successfully completed an NMC validated mentorship programme will need to become a sign-off mentor before assessing any pre-registration student.

There is no specific course available for nurses to become a sign-off mentor, but your organisation, in association with the local university, will have a process in place for you to become a sign-off mentor, taking into account the NMC requirements for becoming a sign-off mentor.

Before you can operate as a sign-off mentor you need to fulfil additional criteria (see box below).

NMC criteria for becoming a sign-off mentor (adapted from NMC, 2008b, page 21)

- Being specifically included on the local database as a sign-off mentor.
- Being registered and working in the same field of practice as the field in which the student intends to register.
- Having clinical currency and capability in the field in which the student is to be assessed.
- Possessing a working knowledge of your student's programme requirements, including practice assessment strategies.
- Understanding of NMC registration requirements and the contribution a sign-off mentor makes to these requirements.
- Understanding of accountability to the NMC which requires a sign-off mentor to justify the decision to pass or fail a student's competencies.
- Meeting NMC supervision requirements before signing off a management student.
- You need to be supervised on three occasions signing off a management student by another sign-off mentor or sign-off practice teacher.

The criteria identified by the NMC to become a sign-off mentor have to be met, but there may be some variation between university organisations as to how the criteria and the three supervised sign-offs of a management student are met.

Meeting NMC requirements to be a sign-off mentor

There are not pre-set time limits for you to make the transition from being a mentor to becoming a sign-off mentor. In fact, in midwifery, all mentors need to meet the sign-off mentor criteria before they are able to mentor midwifery students and it is unclear as to why this is so. Andrews et al. (2010) also point out that providing sign-off mentors may be counterproductive. They suggest that more might be achieved in terms of a student's practice progression by addressing concerns about mentoring nursing students in the earlier stages of their course. It seems unfair to students to leave concerns about mentoring and student assessment until the final practice learning opportunity but these are the NMC requirements at the time of writing.

Activity 8.2: Reflection

Review the NMC criteria for becoming a sign-off mentor on page 101. How do the criteria for becoming a sign-off mentor differ from those required of you to become a mentor? How will you know when you are ready to become a sign-off mentor?

A sample answer can be found at the end of this chapter.

As a prospective sign-off mentor, you need, as part of meeting the NMC additional criteria, to have three supervised signing off experiences with a final practice learning opportunity student. The first two of these can be interactive simulations, but the final one must be with a final practice learning opportunity student, supervised by a sign-off mentor or sign-off practice teacher.

Simulating sign-off scenarios

Simulation is used extensively on nursing programmes and can be a powerful learning strategy which increases a person's confidence and ability to respond to real-life events through interactive and authentic learning scenarios (Wilson et al., 2005; Curtis and Dupius, 2008; Simones, 2008). The use of interactive simulations for prospective sign-off mentors should therefore help them to feel more confident in this new role for final practice learning opportunity students. Simulations can help you as a mentor to prepare for your responsibilities as a sign-off mentor, and can mimic situations that you may well encounter. Providing you with some practice in dealing with common situations that may arise will help you to reflect on past experiences and will also help you to think about how you might handle future situations.

Case study

Anna is a final practice learning opportunity student. She has been your student for the last six weeks and has another six weeks to go in your setting. Anna is very punctual and reliable, and works very hard. The only problem that you feel Anna has is that she doesn't always document the care she has delivered and,

continued opposite...

continued...

when handing over the patients she has been allocated to other team members, she often forgets key aspects relating to her patients. You constantly have to prompt Anna during handover and add information to ensure that all relevant information is communicated to other staff.

Both you and other team members have noticed that Anna doesn't like you prompting her. Her body language reflects her irritation when you contribute additional information.

Activity 8.3: Decision-making

As Anna's sign-off mentor, how would you address this situation?

A sample answer can be found at the end of this chapter.

Addressing issues such as those identified in this case study is not easy but needs to be done to ensure that your student is aware of any issues and has the opportunity to work on their performance. It is rewarding for both you as the mentor and for the student when their performance is improved, and your student becomes a successful member of the practice learning team.

Case study

You meet with Anna in one week's time to give her some formal feedback. You tell Anna that you are pleased that she is making good progress with documenting care and with her handover skills. You also say that she seems more relaxed and seems to take suggestions during your discussions before she has to handover to other staff. Anna is now documenting care as she works with patients rather than leaving it until the end of the shift.

Anna says she feels better and can see now where she was going wrong. She also tells you that she felt she was failing at handover and at looking after her patients when you had to add loads of things in at handover. She tells you she was also frustrated that she felt she would never be as good as all the other trained staff.

Activity 8.4: Reflection

Reflect on the feedback given to Anna and her response. How would you respond to Anna's comment about not feeling as good as the other staff? What would you include when documenting Anna's progress in her practice documentation?

A sample answer can be found at the end of this chapter.

Even if your student responds to your constructive advice it is still important to document all issues and responses to your action plan that you have developed. In this way it is explicit that although there have been issues, they have been addressed and there is a written audit trail of how they have been addressed. Alternatively, if you have documented issues and the student still hasn't quite achieved the desired performance, you can try developing a new action plan in order to assist your student in becoming successful. If by the end of your student's final practice learning opportunity there is no improvement to a satisfactory level of performance, you will have your documentation of events to support your final assessment of the student and these will help to explain how you have made decisions about your student's competence.

If your student doesn't seem to be responding to your proposed action plan or able to achieve the actions you have highlighted with them, it is useful to explore and use the support mechanisms available to you. When a student does not seem to be achieving, this can be a particularly stressful time for you and the student, and may be time-consuming.

Using protected time effectively

Making final assessment of your management student can be quite daunting for mentors. You need to be able to vouch for your student's good character, competence and ability to function as a newly registered nurse, and be accountable for your decisions. These are some of the reasons that the NMC (2008b) requires you to have the equivalent of one hour's protected time per week, per management student. Using this time effectively will help you to make your assessments thoroughly and effectively.

Activity 8.5: Decision-making

How would you use your hour per week of protected time when fulfilling the role of sign-off mentor to a final practice learning opportunity student?

A sample answer can be found at the end of this chapter.

You are not allowed to keep records about students in your setting area because of data protection issues but it will be useful to keep a record of activities you undertake in relation to protected time without including the student's name. This can act as points of reference for you should the student challenge your assessment, and will help you to justify how you made your assessment. Occasionally, some students believe you should have an hour directly with the student each week. It needs to be made clear to the student that the protected time is for you as a mentor, not for the student. You are accountable for the assessment you make of your student and you need to be able to justify how you reached the decision you make about competence.

Accountability as a sign-off mentor

A key question that sign-off mentors ask is: how long will I be held accountable for a student's practice after they qualify? You can only be held accountable for your decision at a specific point in time and, as long as you can justify your decision, your accountability stops there.

Scenario

You have a final practice learning opportunity student, Roy, for whom you are the sign-off mentor. From reading the Ongoing Achievement Record, you identify that punctuality was a problem on several of Roy's previous practice learning opportunities. In addition, several mentors reported that his performance was erratic. On most occasions the reports reflected that Roy worked well as a member of the team but, on occasions, it was reported that he didn't always deliver all care that was required according to the patient's plan of care.

During Roy's second week in your setting, you talk to him about the concerns mentors had in previous practice learning opportunities. Roy admits that he knows he didn't take punctuality seriously at times, and sometimes found it difficult to deliver all the care required for patients in the time available to him. He says he will try harder and wants to work on his time management skills. You talk to Roy about what you will expect during this final practice learning and discuss an action plan with him, stating you will monitor these issues throughout.

At the end of Roy's time with you, you are satisfied that he is competent. There have been no issues in terms of punctuality and he has managed a small group of patients effectively, delivering a good standard of nursing care and managing his time effectively.

Activity 8.6: Reflection

Thinking about the scenario, in terms of accountability, how would you justify your assessment in the light of comments from previous mentors?

A sample answer can be found at the end of this chapter.

As with most aspects of nursing, clear and accurate documentation is vital. Don't worry if you think you haven't enough space to write everything that you want to document in the Ongoing Achievement Record. You can write additional notes regarding discussions and action plans you develop with your student. As long as you clearly date and sign additional paperwork and ask the student to sign it, you can send it to your student's personal tutor for filing in the student file that the university keeps on the student. If you do complete additional documentation about the student, it is useful to make a record that you have sent additional comments directly to your student's personal tutor in the Ongoing Achievement Record so that all parties are aware of this.

The importance of the Ongoing Achievement Record

The Ongoing Achievement Record is a vital document in helping you to make your final assessment of a student, as discussed in the previous scenario. Your judgement can differ from previous mentor assessments but you need to justify why your judgement differs. Some students do seem to take longer than others to reach the required standard of competence. However, your student's previous mentors should have addressed issues and concerns, and if concerns are not resolved, the student should not progress onto the next part of the programme. Unfortunately, for whatever reason, some mentors are reluctant to deal with concerns or are unsure of how to address their concerns. As a sign-off mentor, you need to be fair and objective, taking into account other mentor assessments, whilst not relying too heavily on the assessment of others.

At other times, your student just may not be able to make the transition to managing a group of patients with minimal supervision. This can be very distressing for you and the student, and you will probably need the support of your manager, your peers and the education link lecturer for your setting in helping you to deal with this difficult situation.

What do I need to do to remain as a sign-off mentor?

Once you have achieved the additional criteria necessary to become a sign-off mentor, you remain as a sign-off mentor as long as you fulfil the following requirements:

* you have undertaken an annual mentor update;
* you have mentored a minimum of two students in the previous three years;
* you have undertaken a successful triennial review every three years with your line manager, providing evidence of continuing professional development in relation to mentorship.

As an existing sign-off mentor, you will play a key role in developing new sign-off mentors.

The sign-off mentor role in supervising prospective sign-off mentors

In order for a mentor to become a sign-off mentor they need to undertake two simulated sign-off experiences successfully, and be supervised by an existing sign-off mentor (or sign-off practice teacher) signing off a final practice learning opportunity student.

Activity 8.7: Decision-making

If you were asked to supervise one of the mentors in your setting signing off a final practice learning opportunity student, which elements of this process would you consider you need to supervise?

A sample answer can be found at the end of this chapter.

When supervising another mentor in this process it is really important that you act as a good role model and that you are supportive and approachable towards the mentor. The discussion opportunities with the mentor during this process will allow the mentor to clarify issues that they might have and will help them to continue to develop their mentorship skills.

Chapter summary

Within this chapter you have explored the importance of the sign-off mentor role and have explored the criteria that need to be achieved to become a sign-off mentor. How all mentors contribute to the sign-off process has been highlighted as you are reliant on all mentors for developing a sense of how your student performs on a consistent basis. How a mentor becomes a sign-off mentor has also been addressed as well as how you, as a sign-off mentor, can support other mentors to achieve sign-off status.

Activities: brief outline answers

Activity 8.2 (page 102)

Being a sign-off mentor means that you need to be registered on your local mentor database as a sign-off mentor. Before this can happen you have to meet the NMC requirements. The NMC requirements state that you need to be supervised signing off a management student on three occasions. The first two occasions can involve simulated ways of being assessed which can include objective clinical structured examinations (OSCEs), interactive online simulations or face-to-face simulated scenarios (NMC, 2010c). The third occasion requires you to be peer-assessed by an existing sign-off mentor or sign-off practice teacher actually signing off your final practice learning opportunity student.

As a sign-off mentor you also have to work in the same field (branch) that the student is hoping to register in (NMC, 2010c) and must have an in-depth understanding of the NMC registration requirements, particularly in relation to good character and fitness to practice.

Both mentors and sign-off mentors assess a student's competence, but as a sign-off mentor you have increased accountability and need to review the student's Ongoing Achievement Record. It is important to take into account all previous mentors' accounts about your student so that you can justify your decision to sign off your student as competent.

Feeling ready to go through the process of becoming a sign-off mentor is something only you can know. Undertaking simulated sign-off scenarios will help to prepare you for actually signing off a final practice learning opportunity student for the first time. Following this, the peer support from an existing sign-off mentor/practice teacher when you are doing a final assessment on your management student will also help to reassure you. However, you may feel you want someone to supervise you on a second occasion with a student and you can ask for this to happen if you still feel a little uncertain of your abilities.

Activity 8.3 (page 103)

You may have thought of the following:

It would be useful to reflect on why Anna might be forgetting things. It may well be that she hasn't had opportunities previously to hand over to other team members. Checking the Ongoing Achievement Record may also give you some insight as to whether Anna has had experience in handing over to other staff and whether she has had issues with forgetting to document care previously. There may also be evidence of action plans from other mentors who have had to address this issue, or some indication that Anna doesn't respond well to constructive advice and support.

You would need to talk to Anna about not documenting care, as well as how she doesn't seem to respond very well when you try to help her by prompting her when she forgets key information at the patient handover to other staff.

At such an interview it is useful to begin with the positive aspects of Anna's performance before asking her if there are issues she is having difficulty with in relation to managing a group of patients. If Anna doesn't raise the issues that are of concern to you, you would need to tell her how you find her performance in these aspects of nursing. It is important that you document the interview, including the action plan that you agree with Anna and timescales for reviewing her progress.

If you have identified similar issues from other mentors in the Ongoing Achievement Record, you will need to remind Anna that these are issues that have been identified before.

It is really important that you explain to Anna and document clearly the improvements you are looking for in her performance. You need to be very specific about your expectations as her mentor will give Anna concrete aspects of her performance to concentrate on. It is also useful to ask Anna what help you can give her to help her to achieve.

Your action plan may include the following:

- Anna is to document patient progress so that the plan of care and evaluation reflects the current status of the patient. She also needs to ask you to sign her entries according to NMC requirements (NMC, 2010a).
- Before handing over to other staff Anna needs to practise the handover with you so you can discuss any omissions and add them in before the actual handover.
- Ensure Anna uses the patient's plan of care during handover to make sure she doesn't forget key aspects of care/changes in patient status.
- Progress will be reviewed in one week.

Activity 8.4 (page 103)

You may have included the following in your feedback to Anna:

- Reassure Anna that she isn't expected to be as efficient as a registered nurse who has more experience than her. However, she does need to think about how she can continue to work on developing her skills to ensure she doesn't forget to document or handover key elements of care. It is useful to reassure Anna that practising these skills and taking time to think about what she needs to include at handover will develop her abilities in this area.

In terms of what you would document, you might have included the following:

- You are pleased with Anna's progress and her response to your constructive advice.
- Anna takes time to document care as changes happen to ensure all records are up-to-date.
- You have advised Anna to continue to document care as changes happen and to always take time before she hands patients over to other staff in order to think about what is relevant to include in the handover.
- You have advised Anna that if she continues to work as she has over the last week you will be able to sign off her final competencies at the end of her practice learning opportunity.

Activity 8.5 (page 104)

You may have decided to use this protected time in the following ways:

- Interviews: In addition to the preliminary, intermediate and final interviews you may wish to ensure over your student's practice learning opportunity that you provide formal feedback on a regular basis, especially as your student will have a minimum of 12 weeks in your setting.
- The Ongoing Achievement Record will contain information provided by all of your student's previous mentors. Using some of the protected time it is vital to take time to read the Ongoing

Achievement Record. By reading about your student's progress, you can begin to identify if there have been any particular trends relating to your student's behaviour or performance in practice learning. In addition, there may well be some indication as to how your student responds to constructive advice, and whether they have worked on action plans devised by their previous mentors.

- Taking time to talk to your practice learning manager and other members of the healthcare team will also help to guide you in your overall assessment of the student and how they function as a team member.
- If there are aspects of your student's performance that you are concerned about or that require further development, you may spend some time thinking about how to address issues and how to construct an effective action plan. You may also need to consult with your educational link person for advice on this.
- Students are required to keep a portfolio of their learning in practice and to provide evidence to support their practice achievement. You will need to spend time reading and talking to your student about this evidence so that you can advise the student on how they need to develop their knowledge and reflections.
- As the student is expected to manage a small group of patients, you will need to spend some time each day giving the student feedback on their performance and explaining how they can develop further in terms of managing care.
- Teaching and supervising others is a key element of working as a registered nurse and your student will need to be provided with opportunities to practise these skills in order to develop competence.

This is not an exhaustive list but may give you some ideas of how this time might be spent.

Activity 8.6 (page 105)

You may have included the following in your answer:

An issue has been identified by previous mentors and, although you would hope that it would have been addressed by previous mentors, the student has obviously passed progression point two without successful resolution of the problem. Your judgement is that the student has achieved competence, but you need to document that you were aware of the issues identified by previous mentors, that you discussed these with the student, and developed an action plan that the student fulfilled.

If your documentation did not include reference to those prior issues and no action plan to resolve the issues, your assessment could have been questioned.

Activity 8.7 (page 106)

You may have thought of the following:

It is most likely you will be asked to supervise another colleague within your own setting. It will be useful for you to talk the mentor through the responsibilities of being a sign-off mentor and share your own experiences of signing off final practice learning students. To supervise someone else effectively, you will need to satisfy yourself that the mentor is taking into account all information available to them prior to making their assessment of the student. Ideally, you should check the following elements:

- Be present for the preliminary, intermediate and final interviews.
- Give feedback to the mentor about their discussions with the student and what they have documented about the student.
- Read the student's Ongoing Achievement Record to identify any trends in the student's performance or concerns from previous mentors.
- Discuss with the mentor what they are going to say at the final interview and whether they feel the student has achieved all competencies.
- Complete any documentary evidence used locally to verify you have supervised the mentor and that you are satisfied that they meet the requirements for sign-off mentor status.

You may also have worked with the student yourself or have talked to other colleagues about how the student is coping in their final practice learning opportunity.

Useful websites

www.nmc-uk.org
The Frequently Asked Questions give helpful guidance on the sign-off mentor role.

www.nottingham.ac.uk/practicelearning/mentors
There is a resource on this website that helps prospective sign-off mentors work through the first sign-off simulations.

Chapter 9
Evaluating the practice learning experience

NMC mentor domains and the KSF

This chapter maps to the following NMC mentor domains from the *Standards to Support Learning and Assessment in Practice* (NMC, 2008b) and the NHS Knowledge and Skills Framework.

NMC mentor domains

4. Evaluation of learning

Determine strategies for evaluating learning in practice and academic settings to ensure that the NMC standards of proficiency for registration or recording a qualification at a level above initial registration have been met.

5. Creating an environment for learning

Create an environment for learning where practice is valued and developed that provides appropriate professional and inter-professional learning opportunities and support for learning to maximise achievement for individuals.

6. Context of practice

Support learning within a context of practice that reflects healthcare and educational policies, managing change to ensure that particular professional needs are met within a learning environment that also supports practice development.

8. Leadership

Demonstrate leadership skills for education within practice and academic settings.

NHS Knowledge and Skills Framework
- Communication level 4
- Personal and people development level 4
- Service improvement level 2
- Quality level 2
- Learning and development level 3

Chapter aims

By the end of this chapter you will be able to:

- discuss the importance of evaluation of practice learning for quality assurance purposes;
- understand a variety of strategies that can be used to evaluate the effectiveness of practice learning;
- participate in self and peer evaluation to facilitate personal development and contribute towards the development of practice learning.

Introduction

Case study

Lucy works as a community psychiatric nurse in a mental health setting which takes students at any time during their training. Lucy has always believed her setting to be a good place for practice learning; the students always seem OK and they have never had any negative feedback from the School of Nursing, although the lecturer who is linked with their area very rarely visits. Last month her manager and a teacher completed an educational audit of their setting, which included looking at any previous student evaluations of practice. In their evaluations two of the students had commented that whilst they had enjoyed the placement, they felt that they had not been encouraged to make the most of the learning opportunities that were available. An action plan had therefore been developed which included feeding the comments back to the mentors for discussion.

Initially Lucy was quite upset about the students' comments, saying that she always runs through what opportunities are available during the students' preliminary interview, and if they weren't happy why didn't they raise it whilst they were on practice learning – they had never had any problems before. During the discussion it soon became clear that whilst the opportunities were gone through at the initial interview, nothing was written down for the students to refer to. The mentors had also made an assumption that the students would automatically link the opportunities to the outcomes and proficiencies they needed to achieve. Lucy and her colleagues agreed to map the opportunities against the outcomes and proficiencies as recommended by the auditors. When Lucy's new student arrived this week, she was able to use the mapping document they had developed with the student, and give her a copy to take away for future reference during her practice learning opportunity.

As you have progressed through this book, you will have developed a number of key mentoring skills to help you provide good learning experiences for your students. The next step is to evaluate the effectiveness of the learning experiences you are providing for your students. Students spend 50% of their training in practice with mentors. They give feedback on the effectiveness of the theoretical aspects of their course by evaluating the teaching sessions, modules and the overall programme. In this chapter we will be exploring how you can evaluate the practice learning aspects of the students' training, entering into the world of quality assurance.

In everyday life whenever we make a purchase we have an expectation that the purchase will meet our needs (Quinn and Hughes, 2007). Considering the student allocated to you as a consumer, we will be exploring a variety of approaches that evaluate mentors and the environments mentors and their colleagues provide for their students. We will be focusing on yourself and your area, providing you with an opportunity to measure the effectiveness of learning and assessment in your area and enabling you to participate in self- and peer evaluation to facilitate personal development and contribute towards the development of others (NMC, 2008b). The first section of this chapter will focus on what evaluation is and explore different approaches to evaluating the practice learning opportunity areas and mentors. The later section will focus on self-evaluation, guidance to help prepare you for your triennial review and finally an overview of how the NMC monitors the quality of practice learning.

What is evaluation?

Activity 9.1: Reflection

Take a moment to reflect on the last time you were asked to evaluate something, not necessarily relating to healthcare. Identify what it was you were evaluating, how you were asked to evaluate it and what they wanted to know.

There is no sample answer as this activity is based on your own experiences.

You may have recalled that you had been asked to evaluate the service you had received following a telephone call to your energy supplier or the content of a mandatory study day you recently attended. The way you were asked to evaluate may have included an automated yes/no telephone response or an online questionnaire. They may have been evaluating the clarity of advice given, value for money, speed of response, and whether you would recommend them.

What is evaluation of practice learning?

As a registered nurse you will be very familiar and skilled at evaluating care delivery. In your role as a mentor, the term evaluation is used in the context of the student's practice learning experience. Evaluation is not to be confused with the assessment process as is sometimes the case. Assessment is you assessing what learning has been accrued by the student, measuring achievement of competencies. Evaluation is more of an umbrella term, the origins of which mean the overall 'value' of the learning experience or how 'worthwhile' the practice learning opportunity has been. The process of evaluation involves obtaining feedback from relevant people, reviewing and discussing the feedback and planning action to implement change.

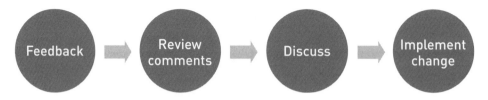

Figure 9.1: The process of evaluation (Kinnell and Hughes, 2010)

Activity 9.2: Critical thinking

Who do you feel should evaluate the students' practice learning experience?

A sample answer can be found at the end of this chapter.

You may have mentioned the student, yourself and possibly the HEI in answer to the above activity. Following basic mentor preparation you are required to continue your development as a mentor, showing at triennial review how you are continuing to meet the domains. The importance of this quality assurance mechanism was highlighted again by the NMC in the Winter 2010 issue of *Update* (NMC, 2010d). By participating in evaluation of practice learning you will be meeting a number of the domain outcomes. Students also have a professional responsibility to evaluate their practice learning experiences, learning how to give honest, constructive feedback. HEIs' approaches to student evaluation of practice learning will vary: some adopt a carrot-and-stick approach and provide incentives to students to complete an evaluation, or punishments to those who don't; for example, withholding the student's next practice learning opportunity details until they have evaluated their previous one. Others take the position that students are adult learners and should be internally motivated and feel that they have a professional responsibility to give feedback to the settings which have supported their learning. Whichever HEI you are attached to, they must ensure that:

- feedback from students and mentors is used to inform the programme and enhance the practice learning experience;
- partners at all levels are committed to and will contribute to quality assurance and enhancement;
- all practice learning experiences are of the same high standard (NMC, (2010a).

How to evaluate the practice learning experience you are providing for your student

Different approaches to evaluating practice learning experiences tend to fall into three categories: educational audit of the practice learning placement, student evaluation of practice learning experiences and mentors' self-evaluation. The following section will provide you with a variety of approaches for use when evaluating the practice learning experience you are providing for your students.

Activity 9.3: Critical thinking

Think for a moment about your place of work. If you were asked to grade your place of work as a learning environment, what score would you give it using 0 = poor and 5 = excellent? List the reasons for the score you have given.

A sample answer can be found at the end of this chapter.

Education audit of practice learning opportunities

In your answer to the previous activity you may have scored your area quite highly and identified that your setting is very prepared for students, that you have a structured programme of learning opportunities and a variety of up-to-date resources. Alternatively, you might feel that your area could be improved and score it lower. This section intends to build on the work you did in Chapter 3 in preparing your learning environment for students. Once you have students allocated to you, as previously mentioned you are audited on a two yearly cycle. As a mentor you have a role in developing the practice learning experience you are providing for your students. Evaluating how effective or ineffective your setting is as a learning environment helps you to fulfil this role. In Chapter 3 you explored how to prepare your learning environment using the key standards. The NMC (2010a) states that: *all practice learning experiences are of the same high standard.* For quality assurance purposes, to avoid any bias, some HEIs ensure that settings are not audited by staff who work in the area or by the education link tutor. What approach to education audits has been implemented by your local HEI?

The next stage, once you have had some students complete an allocation in your setting, is to critically examine your learning environment using the local audit tool, consider what is working effectively, and identify any areas that need to be improved.

Activity 9.4: Leadership and management

Access your placement's last audit document. What are the auditors' recommendations? Has an action plan been developed? If there is an action plan has this been implemented?

There is no sample answer at the end of this chapter as the answer is based on individual experiences.

Some of the most frequently identified recommendations from auditors include:

- the development of a student induction/orientation pack;
- identification of learning opportunities;
- the development of inter-professional learning opportunities;
- mentor updates that need to be completed;
- the development of new sign-off mentors;
- strengthening of links between the university and practice learning opportunity setting.

When completing the previous activity you might have identified that some of the auditors' recommendations have not yet been implemented, or when you looked at the standards you identified additional areas that you feel could be improved. The next step is for you to identify:

- who develops an action plan, if one is required;
- the process for feeding back the outcome of the educational audit to the practice learning opportunity setting;
- who monitors the implementation of the action plan/auditors' recommendations.

Student evaluation of practice

Student evaluations of their practice experience are very useful in informing the auditing process. The auditors will consider the content of the evaluations in preparation for conducting the audit. This enables them to highlight examples of good practice that can be shared with other practice learning opportunity settings and deliver the positive feedback to the staff concerned. It is also an opportunity to identify any reccurring themes that need to be explored further during the auditing process. As mentioned earlier in this chapter all programme providers' quality assurance programmes must ensure that *feedback from students and mentors is used to inform the programme and enhance the practice learning experience* (NMC, 2010a).

The following section explores the processes for ensuring students have the opportunity to evaluate their practice learning experiences. Different HEIs will adopt different approaches to ensure their students are given the opportunity to evaluate their practice learning experiences. Some lecturers will timetable an opportunity for the students to complete their evaluations; others choose to leave it up to the students to complete them in their own time. Some will be online systems and some will be paper-based. As with any type of questionnaire, response rates can be variable, and are often as low as 20%. Generally, HEIs feel that it is very important that students complete their placement evaluations and work towards obtaining a high student response rate by considering different ways to encourage their students to complete them. It is a common responsibility across HEIs for the personal tutor role to include the checking of the student's progress in practice and their overall practice learning experiences, which could involve asking the student if they have completed their evaluation. This might include confirmation in the student's personal academic records and may be completed during end-of-semester tutorials. Ask your educational link tutor how the personal tutor role has been implemented locally to help monitor effectiveness of the learning environments.

> ### Case study
>
> *Tony is a child field student coming up to his first progression point at the end of his first year. He has recently completed his second field-specific practice learning opportunity and has come into the School of Nursing to see his personal tutor. During the tutorial Tony's personal tutor asks him if he enjoyed his last placement. Tony said he had enjoyed the placement, everyone had been really supportive but his mentor had been on annual leave for the first two weeks of his placement then went on a course for two days of his fourth week, so he hadn't really worked much with his mentor. Tony's personal tutor asked him if he had put this feedback in his student evaluation of practice learning (SEPL). Tony said he didn't see the point*
> *continued opposite...*

continued...

> as his mentor had asked him to complete a brief evaluation before he left, which he did. His personal tutor asked him if he had included the issues he had raised in the mentors' evaluation form. Tony said he hadn't as they had all been really nice and supportive.

Activity 9.5: Critical thinking

Why might Tony have decided not to include any negative feedback in his evaluation for his mentor? Consider the advantages and disadvantages of students completing a student evaluation of practice learning opportunity with their mentor.

A sample answer can be found at the end of this chapter.

You may have mentioned that Tony had been reluctant to include negative feedback in his evaluation, as the feedback might have been about his mentor who had given him the evaluation to complete. He might also be concerned that if what he wrote was negative, it could impact on his assessment, or stop him getting a position in that setting when he qualified. For evaluation feedback to be useful it needs to be honest and constructive. Some HEIs choose to anonymise their student evaluations to encourage the students to be honest with their feedback. Do you feel students' evaluations should be anonymous? Does your local HEI anonymise their students' evaluations of practice learning?

Activity 9.6: Critical thinking

Imagine you are a student on a practice learning opportunity. List five questions you feel should be included in your evaluation questionnaire that would measure how good that practice learning opportunity had been.

A sample answer can be found at the end of this chapter.

Below is an example of the questions one HEI has used in their online student evaluation of practice questionnaire. Some of the questions may be the same or similar to the ones you wrote in answer to the previous activity. The format of the questionnaire is a yes/no response and asks for comments to be inserted in a drop-down box.

An example of the questions used in a student evaluation of practice learning questionnaire

1. I was made to feel welcome by the people at the practice learning opportunity area.
2. My orientation was completed by the end of the first week.
3. I was allocated a mentor on or before my first day.
4. I was able to organise my interviews with my mentor.

continued overleaf...

continued...

5. I was able to formulate an action plan with my mentor following my intermediate interview.

6. I was able to develop an action plan following my final interview.

7. I was able to obtain constructive feedback throughout the practice learning opportunity.

8. I was supported effectively by the practice learning opportunity staff/team.

9. I needed additional support during this practice learning opportunity.

   If yes:

   (a) Who did you approach for support?

   (b) Were the issues resolved?

10. The most useful aspects of my practice learning were:

11. My practice learning experience could have been improved by:

Responding to student evaluations of practice learning

The feedback from the students' evaluations should be disseminated back to the settings as soon as is feasible. Interestingly, when giving feedback to practice learning settings regarding responses to these questionnaires, it is common for them to note the number of yes and no responses but it is the comments, the qualitative data, which they tend to focus on and are most interested in. It is also interesting how the evaluations can be full of positive feedback, but if there is one small sentence that is not positive, it will be that particular sentence that is disproportionally focused on by practitioners. For example:

> *This was a wonderful placement, my mentor was brilliant, she really helped me to make sense of how to use evidence to support my practice, it just started to fall into place and has helped my confidence no end. All the staff were helpful and never bothered if I asked questions, if I didn't know something. My mentor was on leave for a week and the place was really busy with winter pressures so I didn't have anyone mentoring me for that week, but I felt I could go to anyone if I needed to.*

However, whilst the majority of student evaluation of their practice learning experiences contain positive feedback, below are some excerpts from completed student evaluations where students have raised particular issues that they were not happy about:

Question: I was made to feel welcome by the placement.

Response: My mentor was really good, and most of the staff were friendly and helpful, but there were two HCAs who seemed to have a problem with students. I don't think they had heard of supernumerary status as at every opportunity they gave me their jobs to do. They made me feel just like a pair of hands rather than a student. I didn't like to say anything to my mentor as she was so nice.

Question: I needed additional support during this placement.

Response: I struggled a bit with my evidence for my portfolio; my mentor tried to help but didn't seem too sure herself. No one from the School visited me and I did try contacting the education link teacher but they were not in.

Activity 9.7: Leadership and management

Select one of the student evaluation comments from the above and write an action plan to address the issue/s raised.

There is no sample answer at the end of this chapter.

The process for the dissemination of the student evaluations back to the settings concerned again will vary across HEIs, but it is often the responsibility of the education link teacher. It would be at this stage that you would need to develop an action plan if either of the above issues had been raised from evaluations. Your action plans for either issue would probably include further exploration of the specifics, like who was involved or should have been involved, informing the ward/setting manager, and identifying specific action to address the problem.

In your own area you might have already come across a student evaluation or attended a staff meeting when student evaluations have been discussed. Identifying your local HEI process for the dissemination of their student evaluation to your setting would be helpful, noting how frequently and how quickly you should be receiving them. If you have not seen any evaluations it would be helpful to ask your education/practice link people if you could see any previous copies or if there is a possibility of viewing any online. If you have not been receiving any student evaluations, identifying the reasons for this would again give you evidence for your triennial review.

It is hugely important that practice learning opportunity settings and mentors receive evaluative feedback, and not only when there is something to address. Mentors invest a great deal of time and effort in supporting students; to receive feedback, especially positive feedback, is very welcome. Initiatives, such as a local annual mentor award, provide students with an opportunity to nominate a mentor who they feel has been particularly effective. One such initiative that has been implemented by an HEI includes a request for nominations on the bottom of their student evaluation of practice form, and this has proved to be quite successful.

Whilst a School-of-Nursing-administered student evaluation of practice provides feedback regarding a number of aspects of a practice learning opportunity, Darling (1985) produced a tool that measures mentorship potential. The development of the measuring mentorship potential tool was based on responses to the questions:

- What do nurses want in a mentor?
- What makes a mentor particularly valuable and helpful?

Three basic mentoring roles were identified from the data: inspirer, investor and supporter. These are then measured within the questionnaire, which you could reproduce or modify as an additional approach to obtain evaluative feedback from your student which is more immediate, although may not be a true and honest evaluation for the reasons previously stated.

Moderating mentors

Whilst it is recognised that assessment of practice learning is not as rigorously moderated as the students' academic work, programme providers are implementing a number of initiatives to help strengthen the inter-mentor reliability. One such initiative involves the moderating of students' practice assessment documentation. A random sample of 10% of the students' practice documentation is moderated by a group comprising lecturers and mentors. The group examine the evidence that the student has provided for the achievement of their competencies. Feedback that is either positive or indicates areas for development is given directly to the mentor concerned by either the education or practitioner link person. The moderating process also provides an opportunity for any particular reccurring themes to be identified and then addressed through the relevant curriculum development groups. You might wish to explore if there are any similar processes happening locally: participating in any such exercise is highly informative and would provide you with evidence to map against the NMC domains in preparation for your triennial review.

Self-evaluation

Evaluating your teaching

As a mentor one area you are responsible and accountable for is facilitating the students' learning using a variety of teaching strategies; in fact, students, it could be argued, are the main consumer of your teaching skills. Whilst the student will be learning from using you as a role model, you are likely to be using informal approaches to facilitating their learning which could involve teaching a skill; for example, assessment of care needs. Once you have delivered the session, obtaining some evaluation feedback from your student regarding your teaching skills would enable you to reflect on this aspect of your mentoring practice, developing your mentoring skills.

Activity 9.8: Critical thinking

You have just delivered a short ten-minute teaching session to your student about record-keeping. Identify five different aspects of your teaching that you would like some feedback on from the student.

A sample answer can be found at the end of this chapter.

You may have asked your student to give you some feedback about how you had delivered the session – was the way you had presented the information clear and easy to understand? Encouraging your student to evaluate your teaching and give you constructive feedback provides you with possible areas for development and evidence for your triennial review to map against the NMC domains. The activity also encourages the student's own development of their skills for delivering feedback and again provides evidence towards achievement of their competencies. So how can you as a mentor implement the proposed changes and developments to your learning environment following an audit or in response to student evaluations?

Mentors as change agents

Implementing auditor recommendations is clearly a collective responsibility of the setting concerned. Change in this instance might be about making small changes to develop the effectiveness of the students' learning experience, a continually unfolding process rather than an either/or event (Sullivan et al., 2009). However, some understanding and application of change theory would be useful to guide, develop and implement the required action plans. You may already have experience of implementing change in your role as a registered nurse; this is where you would be transferring those skills to dealing with practice learning issues.

The first step is to identify what change is needed; that is, what has been recommended by the auditors or identified as action needed following student evaluations of their practice learning opportunity, or what you would like to introduce to improve your students' learning experience. You might, for instance, be interested in developing a learning journey approach to your programme of learning opportunities, or developing more inter-professional learning opportunities for the students. Utilising Lewin's force field model for change (Lewin, 1951) will guide you to identify the driving forces that will help you to implement the change, and the restraining forces, which are those that will impede the change you are suggesting.

Activity 9.9: Critical thinking

Consider a change/development you would like to implement in your area. Identify what might be the driving and restraining forces.

There is no sample answer at the end of this chapter as your response is based on individual experience.

Triennial review

A major element of evaluation and quality assurance processes is the triennial review. The NMC standard to support learning and assessment in practice (NMC, 2008b) requires all service providers to maintain a mentor database/register that contains the details of their active and inactive mentors. All students must have a mentor whose name is on the local mentor database, or be supervised by an associate mentor who themselves are being supervised by a mentor who is on the database. Once you have completed basic mentor preparation your name will be added to your local database. To maintain your live status on the database you are required to undertake a triennial review (every three years). This review is the responsibility of your employing organisation and as such it is usually integrated into current appraisal/development review mechanisms. As part of the review process you must provide your appraiser with evidence of having:

- mentored at least two students within the three-year period;
- participated in annual updating, including an opportunity to meet and explore assessment and supervision issues with other mentors;
- explored as a group activity the validity and reliability of judgements made when assessing practice in challenging circumstances;
- mapped ongoing development in your role against the eight domains;
- been deemed to have met all requirements needed.

Preparing for your triennial review

Most service providers will have developed their own triennial review documentation. It is therefore recommended that you obtain a copy in preparation for your review. This is an opportunity for you to highlight the positive aspects of your mentoring practices. Once you have completed the documentation this will then be kept in your NHS Knowledge and Skills Framework Portfolio (DOH, 2004).

Gathering your evidence

Gathering your evidence for your portfolio should be a continuous process. How you keep data regarding the numbers of students you have supported is up to you. You do, however, need to be mindful of the NMC requirement that *mentors should not keep their own separate student progress records, everything should be contained within the assessment of practice record* (NMC, 2007b). Some settings choose to make a note of mentors and their students on the off-duty records.

As previously mentioned it is an NMC requirement that all mentors attend an annual update to explore curriculum changes and any subsequent impact on the reliability and validity of assessments in practice. Identifying the opportunities that are available for you to update your knowledge is an important step to take. Many of the HEIs that are either supporting or delivering mentor updates have produced registers for you to complete when you attend or complete an update. These registers are then usually forwarded onto the mentor database holder to update their records and for you to access when preparing for your review.

Gathering the evidence that demonstrates your continuing professional development against each of eight NMC domains again should be a continuous process. Recall the different types of evidence that you will have been guiding your students to provide in their portfolios as evidence of their achievement of the competencies.

Activity 9.10: Reflection

Consider for a moment the different types of evidence you can provide that will demonstrate your continuing professional development as a mentor.

A sample answer can be found at the end of this chapter.

You will probably have mentioned feedback from students and reflections on any mentor updates that you might have attended. If you have been using this book for updating purposes, the work you have produced when completing the activities can be used as evidence for your triennial review. Also consider the evidence that you provide for your KSF appraisal to see if it would also be suitable to map against the NMC domains for mentorship.

NMC annual review

Ensuring that triennial reviews have been completed is one of the quality assurance aspects monitored by the NMC during their annual reviews. The final section of this chapter will introduce you to the review process. Whilst undertaking your mentor preparation programme you may have been informed that NMC reviewers visit programme providers to evaluate the quality of the programmes they are delivering. Your placement might have been selected to participate in a previous NMC review. Once the NMC has approved a pre-registration training programme they have a responsibility to annually monitor the quality of those programmes:

> *Risk Based Monitoring is the process by which the NMC is assured that approved programmes continue to be delivered in accordance with NMC standards and additional agreements made at approval.*
> (NMC, 2009)

The NMC seeks to ensure that key risks are controlled by those providing nurse training programmes. They need to know that any weaknesses are addressed in a timely manner and that quality assurance processes (e.g. educational audit, student evaluations of practice learning) are effective in maintaining and enhancing programme delivery in both theory and practice. Programme providers are required to undertake a self-evaluation, currently in the form of an annual report. Self-evaluation is a crucial element of quality assurance and good management; the reviewers will take due account of these evaluations.

The NMC has (in 2011) contracted out the monitoring process to a company called Mott MacDonald who employs the reviewers. The review process requires that a representative sample of practice placements are visited by the reviewers to test how the programme providers control NMC key risks. As a mentor this means that you might be asked to attend a question-and-answer forum where the reviewers ask mentors questions which are focused on the practice learning experiences they are providing for their students.

Once the review has been completed the reviewers award one of the following grades:

- outstanding;
- good;
- satisfactory;
- unsatisfactory.

For each of the following areas:

- resources;
- admissions and progression;
- practice learning;
- fitness for practice;
- quality assurance.

If you would like to know the grades your local programme providers have been awarded, these can be found at www.nmc-uk.org/Educators/Quality-assurance-of-education/Reviewing-and-monitoring/

....

Chapter summary

This chapter has highlighted the importance of effective evaluation of the students' practice learning experience in ensuring the provision of high standard, quality practice learning opportunities for students. The different roles and responsibilities for the evaluation of practice learning have been discussed and analysed. A number of quality assurance processes have also been explored, with opportunities to apply these to your own mentoring practices and the settings where you work as a registered practitioner.

Activities: brief outline answers

Activity 9.2 (page 114)

You may have included some of the following in your answer:

- students;
- school of nursing;
- mentors;
- managers.

Activity 9.3 (page 115)

You may have included some of the following in your answer either positively or negatively depending on the score you gave your workplace:

- high or not so high standards of care;
- new staff are given a good induction;
- study area available/not available;
- resources (e.g. computer facilities, books/journals);
- motivated or de-motivated colleagues;
- staff actively encouraged to develop professionally and personally, or not.

Activity 9.5 (page 117)

You may have included some of the following in your answer:

- advantages – instant feedback, enables you to deal with any issues promptly, honest feedback based on the relationship you have built up with the student, student could use as evidence towards achievement of proficiencies;
- disadvantages – student might be reluctant to give any negative feedback, student may be concerned that what she/he says might influence the mentor who is conducting her/his final assessment.

Activity 9.6 (page 117)

You may have included some of the following in your answer:

- that you had a named mentor;
- that you were made to feel welcome and part of the team;
- that there were lots of learning opportunities;
- that you were encouraged to participate in care;
- that you received regular feedback as to how well you were progressing;
- that your mentor understood what it was you needed to achieve.

Activity 9.8 (page 120)

You may have included some of the following in your answer:

- Was the presentation clear?
- Was it at the right level for the student?
- Was it useful to them?
- Was it interesting?
- Did they feel able to ask any questions?
- Were the resources you used helpful?

Activity 9.10 (page 122)

You may have included some of the following in your answer:

- witness testimonies for students or other colleagues whose learning you may have been supporting;
- work products, which might include a programme of learning opportunities that you have developed for the student;
- evidence that supports evidence based practice and your leadership skills;
- a reflection on an article in a mentors' newsletter or journal that is exploring how to strengthen the reliability or validity of practice assessments;
- a reflection on a discussion you had with your student;
- action plans you may have been involved with following audit or students' evaluations.

Further reading

Royal College of Nursing (2007) *Guidance for Mentors of Nursing Students and Midwives: An RCN Toolkit*, 2nd edn. RCN London.

Useful websites

www.institute.nhs.uk
NHS Institute for Innovation and Improvement.

www.nmc-uk.org
The latest information about the criteria to become a sign-off mentor can be found on this website.

www.nottingham.ac.uk/practicelearning/mentors
An online package is available on this website which can be completed to fulfil the first two simulated sign-off scenarios before being supervised signing off a student in your practice learning setting. There are also some scenarios within the mentor update section that you could utilise to discuss with other mentors some of the common mentoring issues that arise when dealing with students.

www.rcn-uk.org
The RCN Tool Kit that gives guidance to mentors in supporting students and developing the learning environment can be accessed via this web page.

www.nmc-uk.org/Educators
This website provides mentors with information about how the NMC annually monitors all pre-registration nursing and midwifery programmes. It will also enable mentors to look at the results for individual HEIs.

Glossary

Assessment The act of judging someone's competence to undertake activities, sometimes awarding a grade for performance.

Associate mentor A mentor who supports the primary mentor in facilitating learning for a student. However, it may also be a new registrant who has yet to gain a mentorship qualification, who is working alongside a student when the primary mentor is unavailable. Associate mentorship does not involve an assessment role with the student.

Disability A health problem which interferes with an individual's activities of living.

Mentor update Activities which enable a mentor to keep up-to-date with mentorship issues. It should involve discussion elements and involve reflection on mentorship activities. A mentor update has to be undertaken every 12 months for the mentor to remain on the mentor register.

New registrant A description of a newly registered nurse who is currently in their first 12 months of practising as a newly qualified nurse.

NMC reviewers Experienced nursing practitioners or lecturers who are appointed by the NMC's managing body to review the quality of nurse education and/or approve new nursing courses.

Portfolio A commentary of evidence to support the student's learning. It can be presented in a variety of formats and may include a range of evidence that includes some reflection.

Practice teacher A registered nurse or midwife who has undertaken a practice teacher course in order to be able to operate as a stage three mentor. Practice teachers are required for a student undertaking a specialist practitioner qualification.

Preceptorship A period of time following qualification when a new registrant is supported and mentored by an experienced nurse. Preceptorship periods allow the new registrant to consolidate their knowledge and skills whilst working as a registered nurse.

Progression point A point on the nursing education programme where assessment criteria have to be achieved in order for the student to progress onto the next part of their nursing programme. Students cannot continue on their programme until they have met all academic and practice criteria, and this must be achieved within 12 weeks of the progression date. These normally occur at the end of years one and two.

Reflection Activity that involves thinking about experiences, identifying what those experiences mean for those involved in them, and identifying what has been learned or needs to be learned to improve knowledge, skills, attitudes and performance.

Sign-off mentor An experienced mentor who has achieved additional criteria required by the NMC in terms of mentorship. In addition, to become a sign-off mentor the mentor needs to be supervised on three occasions signing off a final placement student and must be annotated on the local mentor database as a sign-off mentor.

Triennial review This is mandatory for all mentors/sign-off mentors and involves a review of mentoring activities by the mentor's line manager. The review needs to be undertaken every three years. The mentor must provide evidence of continued professional development in relation to mentorship, evidence that the individual has mentored at least two students in the previous three years, and evidence that a mentor update has occurred every 12 months.

Work-based learning Learning from experiences which form part of everyday employment activities.

References

Andrews, M and Wallis, M (1999) Mentorship in Nursing: a Literature Review. *Journal of Advanced Nursing*, 29 (1): 201–7.

Andrews, M, Brewer, M, Buchan, T, Denne, A, Hammond, J, Hardy, G, Jacobs, L, McKenzie, L and West, S (2010) Implementation and Sustainability of the Nursing and Midwifery Standards for Mentoring in the UK. *Nurse Education in Practice*, 10 (5): 251–5.

Aston, L and Molassiotis, A (2003) Supervising and Supporting Student Nurses in Clinical Placements: the Peer Support Initiative. *Nurse Education Today*, 23 (3): 202–10.

Aston, L, Wakefield, J and McGown, R (2010) *The Student Nurse Guide to Decision-Making in Clinical Practice*. Milton Keynes: Open University Press.

Atkins, S and Williams, A (1995) Registered Nurses Experiences of Mentoring Undergraduate Nursing Students. *Journal of Advanced Nursing* 21 (5): 1006–15.

Barga, N (1996) Students with Learning Disabilities in Higher Education Managing a Disability. *Journal of Learning Disabilities*, 29: 413–21.

Barlow, S (1991) Impossible Dream. *Nursing Times*, 87 (1): 53–4.

Bartlett, D and Moody, S (2000) *Dyslexia in the Workplace*. London: Whurr.

Benner, P (1984) *From Novice to Expert: Excellence and Power in Clinical Nursing Practice*. Reading, MA: Addison Wesley.

Blankfield, S (2001) Thick, Problematic and Costly? The Dyslexic Student on Work Placement. *Skill*, 70: 23–36.

Bondy, K (1983) Criterion-Referenced Definitions for Rating Scales in Clinical Education. *Criteria in Clinical Evaluation*, 22 (9): 376–82.

Borges, JR and Clement Smith, B (2004) Strategies for Mentoring a Diverse Nursing Workforce. *Nurse Leader*, 2 (3): 45–8.

Brodie, D, Andrews, G, Andrews, J, Thomas, G, Wong, J and Rixon, L (2004) Perceptions of Nursing: Confirmation, Change and the Student Experience. *International Journal of Nursing Studies*, 41 (7): 721–3.

Burnard, P (1988) A Supporting Act. *Nursing Times*, 84 (46): 27–8.

Cowan, D, Norman, I and Coopamah, V (2007) Competence in Nursing Practice: A Controversial Concept – A Focused Review of the Literature. *Accident and Emergency Nursing*, 15 (1): 20–6.

Curtin, MM and Dupuis, MD (2008) Development of Human Patient Simulation Programs: Achieving Big Results with a Small Budget. *Journal of Nursing Education*, 47 (11): 522–3.

Curzon, LB (2003) *Teaching in Further Education: An Outline of Principles and Practice*, 5th edn. London: Cassell.

Darling, LAW (1984) What do Nurses Want in a Mentor? *The Journal of Nursing Administration*, October: 42–44.

Darling, LA (1985) What do Nurses Want in a Mentor? *Nurse Educator*, January–February: 18–20.

Davies, B, Neary, M and Philips, R (1994) *The Practitioner-Teacher: A Study in the Introduction of Mentors in the Pre-registration Nurse Education Programme in Wales*. Cardiff: School of Education, University of Wales.

DOH (2000) *Loooking Beyond Labels: Widening the Employment Opportunities for Disabled People in the New NHS*. London: Department of Health.

DOH (2004) *The NHS Knowledge and Skills Framework (NHS KSF) and the Development Review Process.* London: Department of Health.

DOH and ENB (2001) *Preparation of Mentors and Teachers: A Framework of Guidance.* London: Department of Health and English National Board.

Donaldson, JH and Carter, D (2005) The Value of Role Modelling: Perceptions of Undergraduate and Diploma Nursing (adult) Students. *Nurse Education in Practice,* 24 (5): 353–9.

Downie, C and Basford, P (eds.) (2003) *Teaching and Assessing in Clinical Practice: A Reader.* London: Greenwich University Press.

Driscoll, J (2000) *Practising Clinical Supervision: A Reflective Approach.* Edinburgh: Balliere Tindall in association with the RCN.

Driscoll, J (2007) *Practising Clinical Supervision: A Reflective Approach for Health Care Professionals,* 2nd edn. Edinburgh: Balliere Tindall.

Duffy, K (2004) *Failing Students: A Qualitative Study of Factors that Influence the Decisions Regarding Assessment of Students' Competence in Practice.* Glasgow: Caledonian University.

Earnshaw, GJ (1995) Mentorship: the Student's Views. *Nurse Education Today,* 15: 274–9.

ENB (1989) *Preparation of Teachers, Practitioner/Teachers, Mentors and Supervisors in the Context of Project 2000.* London: English National Board.

Equality Act (2010) *Equality Act 2010: What do I Need to Know? Disability Quick Start Guide.* London: Government Equalities Office.

Evans, W and Kelly, B (2004) Pre-Registration Diploma Student Nurse Stress and Coping Measures. *Nurse Education Today,* 24 (6): 473–82.

Field, D (2004) Moving from Novice to Expert – the Value of Learning in Clinical Practice: A Literature Review. *Nurse Education Today,* 24 (7): 560–5.

Gainsbury, S, Accessed 12/05/2010 at http://www.nursingtimes.net/whats-new-in-nursing/news-topics/health-workforce/me

Gibbons, C, Dempster, M and Moutray, M (2007) Stress and Eustress in Nursing Students. *Journal of Advanced Nursing,* 61 (3): 282–90.

Gibbs, G (1988) Learning by Doing: A Guide to Teaching and Learning Methods. Available at: The Geography Discipline: http://www2.glos.ac.uk/gdn/gibbs/index.htm.

Gonczi, A (1994) Competency Based Assessments in the Professions in Australia. *Assessment in Education,* 1 (1): 27–44.

Gray, MA and Smith, LN (2000) The Qualities of an Effective Mentor from the Student Nurse Perspective: Findings from a Longitudinal Qualitative Study. *Journal of Advanced Nursing,* 32 (6): 1542–9.

Greenwood, J (2000) Critique of the Graduate Nurse: An International Perspective. *Nurse Education Today,* 20: 17–23.

Gunner, A (1988) *Meeting the Future Now: Innovations in Nurse Education.* London: Royal College of Nursing.

Haggerty, B (1986) A Second Look at Mentors: Do you Really Need one to Succeed in Nursing? *Nursing Outlook,* 34 (1): 16–19.

Hart, G and Rotem, A (1994) The Best and the Worst: Students' Experience of Clinical Education. *The Australian Journal of Advanced Nursing,* 11 (3): 26–33.

Harvey, G, Loftus-Hills, A, Rycroft-Malone, J, Titchen, A, Kitson, A, McCormack, B and Seers, K (2002) Getting Evidence into Practice: the Role and Function of Facilitation. *Journal of Advanced Nursing*, 37 (6): 577–88.

Higgins, A and McCarthy, M (2005) Psychiatric Nursing Students' Experiences of Having a Mentor During their First Practice Placement: an Irish Perspective. *Nurse Education in Practice*, 5 (4): 218–24.

Honey, P and Mumford, A (1992) *The Manual of Learning Styles*. Maidenhead: Peter Honey Publications.

Hoong Sin, C and Fong, J (2008) Do no Harm? Professional Regulation of Disabled Nursing Students and Nurses in Great Britain. *Journal of Advanced Nursing*, 62 (6): 642–52.

Ijiri, L and Kudzma, E (2000) Supporting Nursing Students with Learning Disabilities: A Metacognitive Approach. *Journal of Professional Nursing*, 16 (3): 149–57.

Illingworth, K (2005) The Effects of Dyslexia on the Work of Nurses and Healthcare Assistants. *Nursing Standard*, 19 (38): 41–8.

Jarvis, P (2005) Lifelong Education and its Relevance to Nursing. *Nurse Education Today*, 25: 655–60.

Johns, C (2005) *Becoming a Reflective Practitioner*, 2nd edn. Oxford: Blackwell Science.

Kinnell, D and Hughes, P (2010) *Mentoring Nursing and Health Care Students*. London: Sage.

Knapper, CK and Cropley, AJ (1985) *Lifelong Learning and Higher Education*. London: Groom Helm.

Kolb, D. (1984) *Experiential Learning: Experience as a Source of Learning and Development*. Englewood Cliffs, NJ: Prentice Hall.

Konur, O (2002) Access to Nursing Education by Disabled Students: Rights and Duties of Nursing Programmes. *Nurse Education Today*, 22 (5): 364–74.

Levett-Jones, T and Lathlean, J (2008) Belongingness: A Pre-requisite for Nursing Students' Clinical Learning. *Nurse Education in Practice*, 8 (2): 103–11.

Mallik, M and Aylott, E (2005) Facilitating Practice Learning in Pre-registration Nursing Programmes – a Comparative Review of the Bournemouth Collaborative Model and Australian Models. *Nurse Education in Practice*, 5 (3): 152–60.

Marriott, A (1991) The Support, Supervision and Instruction of Nurse Learners in Clinical Areas: a Literature Review. *Nurse Education Today*, 11 (4): 261–9.

Maslow, AH (1970) *Motivation and Personality*. New York: Harper and Row.

McAllister, M (1998) Competency Standards: Clarifying the Issues. *Contemporary Nurse*, 7 (3): 131–7.

McLaughlin, K, Moutray, M and Muldoon, O (2008) The Role of Personality and Self-Efficacy in the Selection and Retention of Successful Nursing Students: a Longitudinal Study. *Journal of Advanced Nursing*, 61 (2): 311–21.

McMullam, M, Endacott, R, Gray, M, Jasper, M, Miller, C, Scholes, J and Webb, C (2003) Portfolios and Assessment of Competence: a Review of the Literature. *Journal of Advanced Nursing*, 41 (3): 283–94.

McMullan, M, Gray, M, Jasper, M, Miller, C, Scholes, J and Webb, C (2003) Portfolios and Assessment of Competence: a Review of the Literature. *Journal of Advanced Nursing*, 41 (3): 283–94.

Melia, K (1987) *Learning and Working: The Occupational Socialisation of Nursing*. London: Tavistock.

Miller, J (2006) Opportunities and Obstacles for Good Work in Nursing. *Nursing Ethics*, http://nej.sagepub.com.cgi/content/abstract/13/5/471. Accessed 8.01.10.

Morris, D and Turnbull, P (2006) Clinical Experiences of Students with Dyslexia. *Journal of Advanced Nursing*, 54 (2): 238–47.

Morris, D and Turnbull, P (2007) The Disclosure of Dyslexia in Clinical Practice: Experiences of Student Nurses in the United Kingdom. *Nurse Education Today*, 27 (1): 35–42.

Myell, M, Levett-Jones, T and Lathlean, J (2008) Mentorship in Contemporary Practice: the Experiences of Nursing Students and Practice Mentors. *Journal of Clinical Nursing*, 17: 1834–42.

Neary, M (2000) *Teaching, Assessing and Evaluation for Clinical Competence: A Practical Guide for Practitioners and Teachers.* Cheltenham: Nelson Thornes.

Newton, A and Smith, LN (1998) Practice Placement Supervision: the Role of the Personal Tutor. *Nurse Education Today*, 18 (6): 496–504.

NMC (2002) *Requirements for Pre-registration Nursing Programmes.* London: Nursing and Midwifery Council.

NMC (2004a) *NMC Principles for Practice Learning for Programmes Leading to Entry on the Professional Register*, QA factsheet c/2004UK. London: Nursing and Midwifery Council.

NMC (2004b) *Requirements for Good Health and Good Character*, Guidance 06/04. London: Nursing and Midwifery Council.

NMC (2004c) *Standards of Proficiency for Pre-registration Nursing Education.* London: Nursing and Midwifery Council.

NMC (2006) *Standards to Support Learning and Assessment in Practice.* London: Nursing and Midwifery Council.

NMC (2007a) Guidance for the Introduction of the Essential Skills Clusters for Pre-registration Nursing Programmes. *Annexe 1 to NMC Circular.* London: Nursing and Midwifery Council.

NMC (2007b) *Nursing and Midwifery Council Circular 33/2007.* London: Nursing and Midwifery Council.

NMC (2007c) *Revised Arrangements for the Introduction of the Practice Teacher Standard in Relation to Specialist Community Public Health Nursing Programmes*, NMC Circular 08/2007. London: Nursing and Midwifery Council; www.nmc-uk.org.

NMC (2008a) *The Code: Standards of Conduct, Performance and Ethics for Nurses and Midwives.* NMC, London.

NMC (2008b) *Standard to Support Learning and Assessment in Practice: NMC Standards for Mentors, Practice Teachers and Teachers*, 2nd edn. London: Nursing and Midwifery Council; www.nmc-uk.org.

NMC (2009) *Quality Assurance Handbook.* Mott MacDonald. Accessed 17.11.2010 at http://www.nmc-uk.org/Educators/Quality-assurance-of-education/Reviewing-and-monitoring/

NMC (2010a) *Education Standards for Pre-registration Nursing Programmes.* London: Nursing and Midwifery Council, online at www.nmc-uk.org.

NMC (2010b) *Record Keeping: Guidance for Nurses and Midwives.* London: Nursing and Midwifery Council, online at www.nmc-uk.org.

NMC (2010c) *Sign off Mentor Criteria*, Circular 05/2010. London: Nursing and Midwifery Council, online at www.nmc-uk.org/documents/circulars.

NMC (2010d) *Update*, Winter 2010. London: Nursing and Midwifery Council.

Norman, IJ, Watson, R, Murrells, T, Calman, L and Redfern, S (2002) The Validity and Reliability of Methods to Assess the Competence to Practice of Pre-registration Nursing and Midwifery Students. *International Journal of Nursing Studies*, 39: 133–45.

Onyett, S (1997) Collaboration and the Mental Health Team. *Journal of Interprofessional Care*, 11 (3): 257–67.

Papp, I, Markannen, M and Von Bondsorff, M (2003) Clinical Environment as a Learning Environment: Student Nurses' Perceptions Concerning Clinical Learning Experiences. *Nurse Education Today*, 23 (4): 262–8.

Pearcey, P and Elliott, B (2004) Student Impressions of Clinical Nursing. *Nurse Education Today,* 24 (5): 382–7.

Quinn, FM and Hughes, SJ (2007) *Principles and Practice of Nurse Education,* 5th edn. Cheltenham: Nelson Thornes.

Rogers, P and Lawton, C (1995) Self Assessment of Project 2000 Supervision. *Nursing Times,* 91 (39): 42–5.

Rowntree, D (1987) *Assessing Students: How Shall we Know Them?* London: Kogan Page.

Ryan, J (2003) Continuous Professional Development along the Continuum of Lifelong Learning. *Nurse Education Today,* 23: 498–508.

Sanderson-Mann, J and McCandless, F (2005) Guidelines to the United Kingdom Disability Discrimination Act (DDA) 1995 and the Special Educational Needs and Disability Act (SENDA) 2001 with Regard to Nurse Education and Dyslexia. *Nurse Education Today,* 25 (7): 542–9.

Schon, D (1983) *The Reflective Practitioner.* New York: Basic Books.

Sheu, S, Lin, H-S and Hwang, S-L (2002) Perceived Stress and Psycho-social Status of Nursing Students During their Initial Period of Clinical Practice: the Effect of Coping Behaviours. *International Journal of Nursing Studies,* 39 (2): 165–75.

Simones, J (2008) Creating a Home Care Simulation Laboratory. *Journal of Nursing Education,* 47 (3): 131–3.

Skingley, A et al. (2007) Supporting Practice Teachers to Identify Failing Students. *British Journal of Community Nursing,* 12 (1): 28–32.

Spouse, J (1996) The Effective Mentor: A Model for Student Centred Learning. *Nursing Times,* 92 (13): 32–5.

Spouse, J (2000) An Impossible Dream? Images of Nursing Held by Pre-registration Students and their Effect on Sustaining Motivation to Become Nurses. *Journal of Advanced Nursing,* 32 (3): 730–9.

Spouse, J (2001) Workplace Learning: Pre-registration Students' Perspectives. *Nurse Education in Practice,* 1 (3): 149–56.

Steinaker, N and Bell, M (1979) *The Experimental Taxonomy.* New York: Academic Press.

Sullivan, EJ and Decker, PJ (2009) *Effective Leadership and Management in Nursing,* 7th edn. Englewood Cliffs, NJ: Prentice Hall.

Walton, J and Reeves, M (1999) *Assessment of Clinical Practice: The Why, Who, When and How of Assessing Nursing Practice.* Wiltshire: Cromwell Press.

Watson, S (2000) The Support that Mentors Receive in the Clinical Setting. *Nurse Education Today,* 20: 585–92.

Watson, S (2004) Mentor Preparation: Reasons for Undertaking the Course and Expectations of the Candidates. *Nurse Education Today,* 24 (7): 30–40.

White, E, Davies, S, Twinn, S and Riley, E (1993) *A Detailed Study of the Relationships Between Teaching, Support, Supervision and Role Modelling for Students in Clinical Areas Within the Context of Project 2000 Courses.* London: English National Board for Nursing, Midwifery and Health Visiting.

Wilson, M, Shepherd, I, Kelly, C and Pitzner, J (2005) Assessment of a Low Fidelity Human Patient Simulator for the Acquisition of Nursing Skills. *Nurse Education Today:* 55–67.

Index